The Vegan Pregnancy Cookbook

OVER 200 RECIPES to keep you and baby
happy and healthy for all three trimesters (and beyond)!

LORENA NOVAK BULL, RD
and **JOLINDA HACKETT**

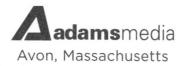

A adamsmedia
Avon, Massachusetts

Published by
Adams Media, a division of F+W Media, Inc.
57 Littlefield Street, Avon, MA 02322. U.S.A.
www.adamsmedia.com

ISBN 10: 1-4405-6075-7
ISBN 13: 978-1-4405-6075-0
eSBN 10: 1-4405-6076-5
eISBN 13: 978-1-4405-6076-7

Printed in the United States of America.

10 9 8 7 6 5 4 3 2 1

Contains portions of material adapted and abridged from *The Everything® Vegan Pregnancy Book* by Reed Mangels, PhD, RD, LD, FADA, copyright © 2011 by F+W Media, Inc., ISBN 10: 1-4405-2551-X, ISBN 13: 978-1-4405-2551-3; *The Everything® Pregnancy Book, 3rd Edition* by Paula Ford-Martin, copyright © 2007 by F+W Media, Inc., ISBN 10: 1-59869-286-0; ISBN 13: 978-1-59869-286-0; and *The Everything® Vegan Cookbook,* by Jolinda Hackett with Lorena Novak Bull, RD, copyright © 2010 by F+W Media, Inc., ISBN 10: 1-4405-0216-1, ISBN 13: 978-1-4405-0216-3.

Always follow safety and commonsense cooking protocol while using kitchen utensils, operating ovens and stoves, and handling uncooked food. If children are assisting in the preparation of any recipe, they should always be supervised by an adult.

This book is intended as general information only, and should not be used to diagnose or treat any health condition. In light of the complex, individual, and specific nature of health problems, this book is not intended to replace professional medical advice. The ideas, procedures, and suggestions in this book are intended to supplement, not replace, the advice of a trained medical professional. Consult your physician before adopting any of the suggestions in this book, as well as about any condition that may require diagnosis or medical attention. The author and publisher disclaim any liability arising directly or indirectly from the use of this book.

Many of the designations used by manufacturers and sellers to distinguish their product are claimed as trademarks. Where those designations appear in this book and F+W Media was aware of a trademark claim, the designations have been printed with initial capital letters.

This book is available at quantity discounts for bulk purchases.
For information, please call 1-800-289-0963.

Contents

CHAPTER 9

Desserts 221

Introduction

Pregnancy is a time of big change for you and family and it's exciting to think about having a new family member. But how can you balance your vegan lifestyle with what's healthy for your baby?

Well, today, more and more women are realizing that a vegan diet is a healthy way to eat during pregnancy and that there's no reason to stop being vegan just because you're pregnant. Still, if you're experiencing or considering a vegan pregnancy you may be feeling a little nervous. You may wonder where you can go to find answers to questions like, "What are some recipes I can try during my pregnancy?," "Am I getting enough protein?," and "How can I ensure that I'm getting the nutrients that I—and my baby-to-be—need?" Fortunately, *The Vegan Pregnancy Cookbook* is here to answer your questions and keep you healthy and happy for the duration of your pregnancy and beyond. Here you'll find more than 200 delicious, vegan recipes each with nutrient icons (described in Part 2) designating the amount of folic acid, vitamin B_{12}, protein, and so on that each recipe contains to help you learn which recipes to put together during the day to keep your nutrient intake consistent and safe for you and your baby-to-be. The recipes—ranging from breakfasts to appetizers to desserts—will give you lots of ideas and opportunities to try new foods and vegan versions of some favorite dishes. You'll also find information on how you can eat a balanced diet; which foods to limit; how to plan out your meals; and which minerals, vitamins, and other nutrients you need to keep your baby's growth on track.

So get ready to eat healthfully during your vegan pregnancy. After all, no one said that eating vegan couldn't be delicious—and good for you and your baby-to-be! Enjoy!

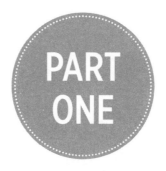

PART ONE

Vegan Nutrition

Whether you've been vegan for many years, are a relative new-comer to veganism, or are simply contemplating being vegan, adding pregnancy to the equation may raise questions. Rest assured, the American Dietetic Association (ADA) has said that well-planned vegan diets are "appropriate for all stages of the life cycle including pregnancy and lactation." Pregnancy (or prepregnancy) is a great time to learn more about vegan nutrition so you can be sure you are making the best possible food choices. Part 1 will show you what you need to be eating and which nutrients, minerals, and vitamins you need to eat throughout your pregnancy.

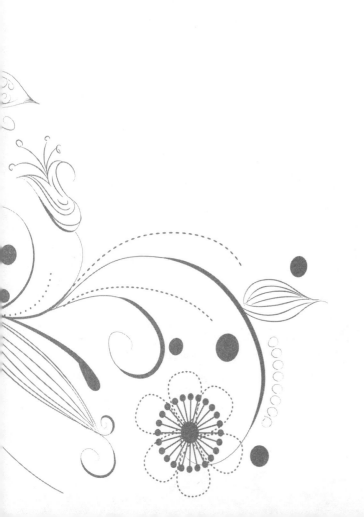

CHAPTER 1

What You Should Be Eating: Vitamins, Minerals, and Other Nutrients

When you're a vegan, there are no specific requirements as to how much (or how little) cooking you will need to do. Some vegans love to prepare meals and create new recipes. Others rely on takeout, convenience foods, and quick-to-fix meals. But no matter how much cooking you decide to take on, during your pregnancy you need to make sure that you're eating the correct amounts of certain nutrients every day to ensure that your baby is developing in an appropriate manner. Fortunately, the key to a nutritionally sound vegan diet is actually quite simple. Eating a variety of foods including fruits, vegetables, plenty of leafy greens, whole-grain products, beans, nuts, and seeds in sufficient quantities virtually ensures that you'll meet most of your nutrient needs, such as vitamins A and C. For the few remaining nutrient needs that can be a bit trickier to meet with a vegan diet, you will need to approach meal planning with a little extra care to make sure that appropriate foods are included to satisfy those needs. Read on to see what you need to be eating during your pregnancy.

Folic Acid

Folic acid (folate) significantly lowers your baby's risk of developing neural tube defects (birth defects of the brain and spinal cord, such as spina bifida and anencephaly). Because the neural tube forms during the first four weeks of pregnancy, before many women even realize they are pregnant, the U.S. Centers for Disease Control (CDC) recommends that *all* women of childbearing age do one of the following:

- Take a vitamin that has folic acid in it every day. This can either be a folic acid supplement or a multivitamin. Most multivitamins sold in the United States have 400 micrograms of folic acid, the amount nonpregnant women need each day. Check the label of the vitamin to make sure that it contains 100 percent of the daily value (DV) of folic acid.
- Eat a bowl of breakfast cereal that has 100 percent of the DV of folic acid every day. Check the label on the side of the cereal box for one that has "100 percent" next to "folic acid."

Use of a vitamin or a breakfast cereal containing 100 percent of the DV for folic acid are both reliable ways to ensure adequate folic acid intake before pregnancy. During the first three months of pregnancy, 400 micrograms of folic acid per day is still adequate; however, you should trade your multivitamin for prenatal vitamins, which provide higher amounts of certain nutrients that are critical in your baby's development. The requirement for folic acid during months 4 through 9 increases to 600 micrograms per day. Check the amount of folic acid in your prenatal vitamin so you will know how much you need to get from the foods that you eat each day. Folic acid is added to breads, cereal, pasta, rice, and flour and is found naturally in leafy dark-green vegetables, citrus fruits and juices, and beans. You may only need small amounts of folic acid, but don't forget it's an essential vitamin. Because the amounts in foods vary and it may be hard to get all of the folic acid you need from food sources alone, be sure to take your prenatal vitamins as recommended by your physician.

Vitamin B$_{12}$

Since vegans must get vitamin B$_{12}$ from fortified foods or supplements, it's important to make sure that you are choosing foods or a vitamin pill that provides this essential nutrient. Vitamin B$_{12}$ plays an important role in the development of the baby's brain and nervous system. Be aware that some foods once thought to naturally contain vitamin B$_{12}$, such as sea vegetables and fermented foods, often contain unreliable or unusable forms of this vitamin called, "B$_{12}$ analogues." Instead, select foods that have been fortified with vitamin B$_{12}$. Foods that may be fortified with vitamin B$_{12}$ include:

- Soymilk, rice milk, and other commercial plant milks
- Meat analogues (veggie "meats")
- Breakfast cereals

- Energy bars and protein bars
- Marmite yeast extract
- Tofu
- Nutritional yeast

Before you are pregnant, you need 2.4 micrograms of vitamin B_{12} daily; once you're pregnant, the daily reference intake (DRI) increases to 2.6 micrograms. A food or supplement that contains at least 45 percent of the DV for vitamin B_{12} will provide enough to meet these needs. One easy way to make sure you're getting enough of this vitamin is to take a daily multivitamin that provides at least 45 percent of the DV for vitamin B_{12}.

Protein

Proteins are responsible for everything from the structure of your muscles and bones to the proper function of your immune system to food digestion. In pregnancy, extra protein is needed to support your baby's growth—building bones and muscles, for example. You also need extra protein as your blood volume increases and your breasts and uterus enlarge.

Before you were pregnant, you needed around 0.4 grams of protein for every pound that you weighed. The math isn't hard to do. Take your prepregnant weight in pounds and multiply by 0.4—that's how much protein you needed before you were pregnant. For instance, if you weighed 120 pounds, you'd multiply 120 by 0.4 and get 48 grams of protein. The first trimester of pregnancy, you actually don't need any more protein than this because your baby is so small and your body changes are less than they will be later on.

Starting with the fourth month of pregnancy, protein needs increase to support changes to your body and your baby's growth. You need about 25 grams of protein a day more than you did before you were pregnant or in the first trimester. Simply take the amount of protein recommended before pregnancy (0.4 times your prepregnant weight) and add 25. That's how much daily protein (in grams) is recommended. This amount is about 50 percent higher than protein recommendations for nonpregnant women. So for instance, if you weighed 120 pounds before pregnancy, you'd multiply 120 by 0.4 and then add 25 for a total of 73 grams of protein. However, if math makes your head spin, feel free to use the general protein recommendation for pregnant women during the second and third trimesters, which is 71 grams per day.

Foods that provide protein include all varieties of beans from adzuki to yellow beans, grains, nuts and seeds, nut butters and seed butters, vegetables, potatoes, soy foods, meat analogues (products made to resemble meats), tempeh, lentils, and seitan (wheat "meat"). Most of these foods have 20 or more grams of protein in a serving—a cup of beans or 4 ounces of tempeh. Other foods that provide generous amounts of protein (10–20 grams per serving) include tofu, veggie burgers, and cooked dried beans. Soymilk, peanut butter, soy yogurt, and quinoa are all good sources of protein as well. Vegetables, whole grains, pasta, almond butter, and nuts and seeds are other good foods to add to your protein intake.

Iron

Iron's major role is to help red blood cells deliver oxygen throughout your body. When you are pregnant, iron also helps deliver oxygen to your baby. In pregnancy, your body's blood supply actually increases 40–50 percent. In order to make this extra blood, you need more iron than you do when you're not pregnant. Your unborn baby is also storing iron that will meet her needs for the first few months of life outside your womb. Baby takes what she needs from your store of iron first, so she won't suffer unless you are very low in iron. However, you can end up with iron-deficiency anemia.

It's possible, with smart food choices, for vegan women to meet the DRI for non-pregnant women of 18 milligrams of iron per day and 27 milligrams per day for pregnant women. While many of the foods vegans eat supply iron, the following foods are some of the highest sources:

- Iron-fortified breakfast cereals
- Cream of Wheat or instant oatmeal
- Tofu
- Blackstrap molasses
- Iron-fortified energy bars
- Soybeans
- Dark chocolate
- Lentils
- Spinach
- Chickpeas

When you add in the higher iron needs that go with pregnancy, however, many women find that taking a daily iron pill, along with choosing high-iron foods, is what they need. Did you know that foods high in vitamin C will enhance the absorption of iron from both food and supplements when consumed together at the same meal? Try topping a bowl of iron-rich beans with fresh tomato salsa, or swallow your iron supplement with a glass of orange juice. On the other hand, both calcium and caffeine inhibit iron absorption, so avoid drinking caffeinated or calcium-fortified beverages with your supplements and foods that are high in iron. So if you take your iron pill with orange juice, be sure to use juice that is not fortified with calcium.

Zinc

Zinc plays an important role in your baby's development, so it's a mineral to be aware of. Zinc requirements go up with pregnancy. Coincidentally, the amount of zinc that you absorb from meals increases also. Some breakfast cereals are fortified with zinc, as are some veggie "meats" and energy bars. If you're looking for higher zinc brands, check the Nutrition Facts label at the grocery store. Adding a spoonful or two of wheat germ to hot cereals or other grain dishes provides extra zinc. Vegetables that have the highest amounts of zinc include mushrooms, spinach, peas, corn, and asparagus. Fruits are not an especially good way to get zinc. Dark chocolate is not just a good way to get iron, but it also provides zinc—and has more of either of these minerals than does milk chocolate. The DRI for zinc is 11 milligrams per day. The following vegan foods are especially good zinc sources:

- Zinc-fortified breakfast cereals (up to 15 milligrams of zinc in 1 ounce of cereal)
- Wheat germ (2.7 milligrams in 2 tablespoons)
- Zinc-fortified veggie "meats" (up to 1.8 milligrams in 1 ounce)
- Zinc-fortified energy bars (up to 5.2 milligrams in a bar)
- Adzuki beans (4 milligrams in 1 cup)
- Tahini (1.4 milligrams in 2 tablespoons)
- Chickpeas (2.4 milligrams in 1 cup)
- Black-eyed peas (2.2 milligrams in 1 cup)
- Baked beans, canned (5.8 milligrams in 1 cup)
- Peanuts, peanut butter (close to 2 milligrams in 2 tablespoons)

Calcium

Throughout your pregnancy, the calcium from the foods you eat will move from your intestines, into your blood, through the placenta, and to your baby. Although your baby's bones are growing throughout pregnancy, the last trimester is peak growth time. During that trimester, he'll need 200–250 milligrams of calcium a day—a little less than the amount of calcium in a cup of fortified soymilk (if you absorbed all of that calcium). Since you only absorb a third or less of dietary calcium, the DRI for calcium is higher than 200–250 milligrams.

While many foods vegans eat supply calcium, the following foods are some of the highest sources:

- Calcium-fortified plant milks
- Dried figs
- Tofu (especially prepared with calcium sulfate)
- Collard greens
- Kale
- Turnip greens and bok choy
- Calcium-fortified orange juice
- Blackstrap molasses
- Soybeans
- Okra

With pregnancy, calcium needs are higher in order to maintain your bones and to supply calcium for your baby's bone and teeth development. Remarkably, your body compensates for the increased calcium needs by pumping up the amount of calcium that you absorb from your food. Early in pregnancy, the amount of calcium you absorb doubles; higher calcium absorption continues throughout your pregnancy. Since calcium absorption is so high in pregnancy, the recommendation for how much calcium you need doesn't increase above what it was prepregnancy, which is 1,000 milligrams per day. So if you were getting the amount of calcium that you needed before you were pregnant and you're eating similar foods now, chances are good that you're meeting your calcium needs.

Vitamin D

Vitamin D is known as the sunshine vitamin because your body makes vitamin D when your skin is exposed to the sun. Vitamin D is needed for your body to absorb calcium, so it is often linked to healthy bones. Look to fortified foods and supplements for most of your vitamin D needs. Vitamin D is added to many brands of plant milks, including almond milk, hemp milk, coconut milk, rice milk, and soymilk. Some brands of dairy lookalikes (like yogurt and cheese) also have vitamin D added. Breakfast cereals, juices, and energy bars are some other products often fortified with vitamin D.

Fresh mushrooms, identified on the label as being a good source of vitamin D, have been exposed to ultraviolet light that stimulated the mushroom's production of vitamin D. A 3-ounce serving of these mushrooms has about 400 IU of vitamin D or about two-thirds of the recommended daily intake. Vitamin D supplements are another option. Many calcium supplements also contain vitamin D and so do most prenatal supplements. Vitamin D needs do not increase in pregnancy. The RDA for vitamin D in pregnancy is 600 IU, the same as for nonpregnant women. As too much vitamin D can be toxic, before taking extra vitamin D (beyond what is in your prenatal vitamin), check with your health care provider or registered dietitian (RD) to make sure you're not over-doing this vitamin.

DHA

Docosahexaenoic acid (DHA) is a fatty acid most commonly found in the oil from fish. DHA, categorized as an omega-3 fatty acid, plays a role in the development of your baby's vision. DHA may also affect your baby's cognitive development.

In the last trimester, the fetus stores DHA in her brain and in her retina (a part of the eye). If your diet is low in DHA, stored DHA from your body will be used to meet your fetus's needs. Some experts fear this will make your stores of DHA too low. When it comes to DHA, vegans can get some DHA indirectly by taking another omega-3 fatty acid called ALA that is converted to DHA. However, the conversion of ALA to DHA in the body appears to be very inefficient. The best vegan source of DHA occurs in foods and supplements containing DHA that is derived from algae. If you are interested in finding foods with vegan DHA, check the ingredient listing for DHA microalgal oil. Not all foods that contain DHA algal oil are vegan; the oil is also added to some brands of cow's milk, yogurt, and other nonvegan products. Some prenatal supplements contain vegan DHA. Again, check for microalgal oil on the ingredient list. Separate vegan DHA supplements are also available. Although current studies of the function and benefits of

DHA overwhelmingly suggest the need to establish a daily reference intake, or DRI, for for this important nutrient, there presently is none. However, consuming foods containing DHA, or taking a vegan DHA supplement, a couple of times each week may be beneficial.

Iodine

Iodine, a mineral that you may have heard of because it is added to iodized salt, is essential for the development of your baby's brain. Worldwide, iodine deficiency in pregnancy and early childhood is the single most important preventable cause of brain damage. Iodine requirements are higher in pregnancy to make sure your baby gets enough iodine for brain development.

Generally, the need for iodine can be easily met through the use of iodized salt; however, if you don't use much iodized salt, or if you use sea salt or other noniodized salt, you may need an iodine supplement. Many prenatal supplements contain iodine, but not all do. The American Thyroid Association recommends that pregnant women take a daily prenatal vitamin that contains 150 micrograms of iodine. You can get some iodine from your foods; however, the amount of iodine present in plant foods is very small and is sadly unreliable as it is dependent upon the iodine content of the soil in the region in which the vegetables are grown. Sea vegetables like nori and kombu can provide some iodine, but those amounts are also variable. Some sea vegetables are actually very high in iodine, such as arame, hijiki, and kombu, but because excess iodine can cause health problems for you and your baby, you should limit use of these high-iodine sea vegetables during pregnancy.

A Healthy Vegan Diet

Hopefully, you can see that, by making smart food choices, it's easy to eat a healthy vegan diet—one that's good for you, for your baby-to-be, and for the planet. But, before we get to the recipes, let's take a look at how to put all of this information together and how to ensure that you're getting what you—and your little one—need to be healthy.

CHAPTER 2

Vegan Food Guide

You've heard it before—whole grains, beans, fruits, vegetables, and nuts are the basis for a healthy vegan diet. But maybe that's not enough. How many servings of vegetables should you be eating now that you're pregnant? Are there foods that you should avoid? A simple vegan food guide for pregnancy can help. And if you'd like even more support, a session with a knowledgeable registered dietitian (RD) is a very worthwhile undertaking. The RD is the nutrition expert!

Vegan Food Guide for Pregnancy

Many food guides don't work for vegans. Food guides often include a meat group and a dairy group and even if you replace meat with vegetable protein sources, you're still left with a food group that recommends eating cheese and drinking cow's milk.

This vegan food guide for pregnancy is based on five food groups. All servings listed are the minimum number of servings from each food group. If you are not gaining weight at the recommended rate, you'll need to eat a larger number of servings from the food groups. Be sure to choose a variety of foods from each food group.

Recommended Daily Food Choices for Vegan Pregnancy

Food Group	Daily Serving
Grains	6
Dried Beans, Nuts, Milks, and Other Protein-Rich Foods	7
Vegetables	4
Fruits	2
Fats	2

In addition to making food choices based on this food guide, you should also be taking a prenatal supplement that supplies vitamins and minerals including iron, zinc, iodine, vitamin B_{12}, and vitamin D. Supplemental DHA is also recommended in pregnancy.

Grain Group

The grain group includes breads, tortillas, crackers, bagels, rolls, pastas, rice, cereals, quinoa, and other foods made from grains. Choose whole grains often. A serving from this group is a slice of bread; a tortilla or roll; ½ cup of cooked cereal, grain, or pasta; or 1 ounce of ready-to-eat cereal. This food group provides carbohydrates, calories, fiber, B vitamins, iron, and some protein. Fortified cereals can supply other vitamins and minerals.

Dried Beans, Nuts, Milks, and Other Protein-Rich Foods Group

This food group includes a variety of foods that are good sources of protein for vegans. Many foods in this group also supply iron and zinc and some foods are fortified with calcium, vitamin D, and vitamin B_{12}. A serving from this group is ½ cup of cooked dried beans or peas; ½ cup of tofu, TVP, or tempeh; 1 ounce of veggie "meat"; 2 tablespoons of nut or seed butters; ¼ cup of nuts or soy nuts; or 1 cup of fortified soymilk.

Vegetable Group

This food group includes all vegetables, from asparagus to zucchini. Vegetables can be eaten raw or cooked. A serving from this group is ½ cup of cooked vegetables or 1 cup of raw vegetables. Be sure to include some nutrient-rich dark-green vegetables and deep-orange vegetables often. Dark, leafy greens such as kale are a great plant source of calcium. This food group is an especially good source of fiber and vitamins A and C; it supplies some iron and zinc.

Fruit Group

Fruits are especially good sources of vitamins C and A; they also provide fiber and B vitamins. The fruit group includes fresh, frozen, canned, and dried fruits and fruit juices. A serving from this group is a piece of medium fruit; ½ cup of cut up or canned fruit; ¼ cup of dried fruit; or ½ cup of fruit juice.

Fats Group

This group provides calories, vitamin E, and essential fatty acids. Foods in this group include oils, vegan salad dressings and mayonnaise, margarine, and vegan cream cheese. A serving of any of these foods is 1 teaspoon.

Menu Planning

Many women choose to eat three meals and several snacks during pregnancy to stave off hunger pangs and to keep from feeling uncomfortably full as the baby gets bigger. Remember, snacks don't have to be a big production. A piece of fruit and some nuts or trail mix can be a satisfying snack.

Here's a sample menu based on the Vegan Food Guide:

Breakfast
- ½ cup oatmeal (1 serving grains)
- 2 tablespoons almond butter (1 serving protein; calcium source)
- 4 ounces calcium-fortified orange juice (1 serving fruit; calcium source)

Midmorning Snack
- ½ bagel (1 serving grains)
- ½ cup hummus (1 serving protein; calcium source)

Lunch
- Sandwich with 1 slice whole-wheat bread (1 serving grains), 1 ounce vegan deli slices (1 serving protein), and 1 teaspoon vegan mayonnaise (1 serving fats)
- 1 cup mixed greens (1 serving vegetables)
- Medium apple (1 serving fruit)

Midafternoon Snack

- ¼ cup cashews (1 serving protein)
- 1 cup baby carrots (1 serving vegetables)

Dinner

- 1 cup pasta with tomato sauce (2 servings grains)
- ½ cup veggie burger crumbles (1 serving protein)
- ½ cup chickpeas (1 serving protein)
- 1 cup steamed collards (2 servings vegetables; calcium source) with 1 teaspoon olive oil (1 serving fats)

Bedtime Snack

- 1 ounce ready-to-eat cereal (1 serving grains)
- 1 cup calcium-fortified soymilk (1 serving protein; calcium source)

You'll probably need to add some more foods in order to support weight gain. This sample menu shows how to meet the minimum number of servings for the Vegan Food Guide. Be sure to choose a variety of foods and use a daily prenatal supplement.

The Best Foods

Eating a variety of foods is always good advice. That way, if one food that you eat is high in vitamin X but low in mineral Y, you're likely to choose another food that will be low in vitamin X but high in mineral Y. Eating a variety of foods lets you relax and not have to worry about keeping track of every nutrient.

Certain foods in each food group are especially good sources of a variety of nutrients. For example, in the grains group, whole grains supply more fiber and more of some vitamins and minerals than do their refined counterparts. In the vegetables group, dark-green vegetables and deep-orange vegetables are your best choices. That doesn't mean iceberg lettuce and mushrooms are off limits, just that these less nutrient-rich foods should be balanced with some carrots and kale. Fresh fruits provide more fiber than more processed fruits or juices. If you choose to use canned fruits, select fruits packed in fruit juice rather than in heavy syrup. Dried beans, tofu, tempeh, soymilk, nuts, and nut butters are excellent choices from the protein-rich foods group. More processed foods like veggie "meats" are often higher in sodium, lower in fiber, and more expensive.

Foods to Limit

Everything in moderation is a standard piece of nutrition advice. While moderation is a reasonable approach to eating, make sure that you know what "moderation" means. Moderation means that after you have eaten the appropriate amounts of nutrient-rich foods, it's all right to have a small (emphasis on small!) amount of what are often called junk foods.

Junk foods are foods that you would be just fine, nutritionally speaking, if you never ate them again. The sole nutritional value of these foods is that they provide calories; they're not great sources of protein, vitamins, minerals, or other things you need. Examples of junk foods are soft drinks, candy, cookies, cake, chips, and greasy snack foods. Remember, just because a food is vegan doesn't mean it's healthy. What's wrong with these foods? Think of your eating plan like your household budget—you have to make choices to stay on your budget. If you need a certain amount of calories to support weight gain in pregnancy, you don't want to "spend" those calories on non-nutritious foods. Rather, you want to get the best nutrition possible within your allotted calories. If you overdo junk foods, they can displace healthier foods in your diet—not good for you or your baby. That said, if gaining enough weight is a struggle, judicious use of junk foods can help. Once you've eaten your day's share of healthy foods, you can add calories with some higher calorie, lower nutrient foods.

So now that you know what you should—and shouldn't—be eating, let's take a look at the vegan recipes that will help you get the vitamins, minerals, and other nutrients you need!

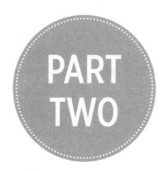

PART TWO

Healthy Recipes for a Vegan Pregnancy

Are you ready to cook and nourish yourself and your baby-to-come with delicious, nutritious vegan meals? You are about to savor a mouthwatering collection of dishes from appetizers to desserts that you are going to love! The keys to good nutrition during a vegan pregnancy, as with any pregnancy, are to consume a carefully selected and varied diet in sufficient quantities to support the growth of the baby and to maintain the health of the mom, with special attention given to nutrients that are sometimes difficult to obtain on a vegan diet. The recipes on the following pages are designed to be chockfull of super-healthful, nutrient-dense ingredients like collard greens, sweet potatoes, tofu, mushrooms, and beans to help you receive those hard-to-get nutrients.

This book has a simple-to-use feature that makes it a snap to find recipes that are high in specific nutrients to meet your personal needs. For example, if at any time during your pregnancy you experience an issue with iron-deficiency anemia, you will be able to flip through the pages and immediately identify dishes that are high in iron! To ensure that you are getting the best possible nutrition, whenever possible, utilize ingredients that are fortified with nutrients like calcium, vitamin B_{12}, and iron. And don't forget to take your prenatal vitamins as prescribed by your physician. Even the most perfectly executed meal plan could be lacking in some vital nutrient due to a variety of causes, including vegetables grown in nutrient-deficient soil.

To help you ensure that your meals contain a sufficient amount of the vitamins and nutrients outlined in the first chapter, you'll find icons at the beginning of each recipe. These icons will help you determine which recipes are higher in various nutrients (up to about 30% of the daily requirement) so you can plan your meals accordingly. One icon represents approximately 2–10% of the daily requirement for a particular nutrient present in one serving of the recipe. Similarly, two icons indicates that one serving provides approximately 11–20% of the daily requirement and three icons indicates that one serving provides approximately 21–30% (and sometimes more!) of the daily requirement for that nutrient. In instances where one serving of a recipe contains less than 2% of the daily requirement you will see a statement indicating that the nutrient is "only present in very small amounts." You will find a similar statement when 100% of the daily requirement for a given nutrient is provided by one serving of a recipe.

While iodine and DHA are both important nutrients, they are not included in this ranking system because food sources of iodine other than iodized salt are unreliable and, as was mentioned in Chapter 1, there is no established daily requirement for DHA. Follow the recommendations in Chapter 1 for iodine and DHA.

The icons will be divided up as follows for the remaining nutrients:

Folic Acid

Note: You want to receive 600 micrograms of folic acid each day.

🍎	12–60 mcg
🍎🍎	61–120 mcg
🍎🍎🍎	121–180 mcg

Vitamin B$_{12}$

Note: You want to receive 2.6 micrograms of vitamin B$_{12}$ each day.

🍎	0.1–0.2 mcg
🍎🍎	0.3–0.5 mcg
🍎🍎🍎	0.6–0.8 mcg

Protein

Note: You want to receive 71 grams of protein each day.

🍎	1–7 g
🍎🍎	8–14 g
🍎🍎🍎	15–21 g

Vitamin D

Note: You want to receive 600 International Units of vitamin D each day.

🍎	12–60 IU
🍎🍎	61–120 IU
🍎🍎🍎	121–180 IU

Iron

Note: You want to receive 27 milligrams of iron each day.

🍎	0.5–2.7 mg
🍎🍎	2.8–5.4 mg
🍎🍎🍎	5.5–8.1 mg

Zinc

Note: You want to receive 11 milligrams of zinc each day.

🍎	0.2–1.1 mg
🍎🍎	1.2–2.2 mg
🍎🍎🍎	2.3–3.3 mg

Calcium

Note: You want to receive 1000 milligrams of calcium each day.

🍎	20–100 mg
🍎🍎	101–200 mg
🍎🍎🍎	201–300 mg

So what are you waiting for? It's time to get cooking!

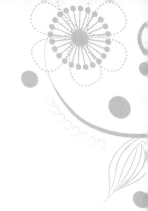

CHAPTER 3

Vegan Breakfasts

Carob-Peanut Butter-Banana Smoothie

Yummy enough for a dessert but healthy enough for breakfast, this smoothie is also a great protein boost. Grab a whole-grain muffin and you have breakfast to go.

SERVES 2

7–8 ice cubes

2 bananas

2 tablespoons peanut butter

2 tablespoons carob powder

1 cup fortified soymilk

Folic Acid:

Vitamin B$_{12}$:

Protein:

Iron:

Zinc:

Calcium:

Vitamin D:

Place all ingredients in a blender and blend together until smooth.

Per Serving
Calories: 262 | Fat: 10g | Sodium: 136mg | Fiber: 6g | Protein: 9g

Strawberry Smoothie

If you're craving fruit during your pregnancy, this is a great way to start your day. Add silken tofu to a simple fruit smoothie for a creamy protein boost.

SERVES 2

½ cup frozen strawberries
(or other berries)

½ (16-ounce) block silken tofu

1 banana

¾ cup orange juice

3–4 ice cubes

1 tablespoon agave nectar
(optional)

Folic Acid: 🍎

Vitamin B$_{12}$: NA

Protein: 🍎

Iron: 🍎

Zinc: 🍎

Calcium: 🍎

Vitamin D: NA

- Place all ingredients in a blender and blend together until smooth and creamy.

Per Serving
Calories: 154 | Fat: 3g | Sodium: 6mg | Fiber: 3g | Protein: 5g

Vanilla-Date Breakfast Smoothie

Adding dates to a basic soymilk and fruit smoothie adds a blast of unexpected sweetness. This recipe works as either a healthy breakfast treat or as a cooling snack for the times when those pregnancy hot flashes hit.

SERVES 1

4 dates

Water

¾ cup fortified soymilk

2 bananas

6–7 ice cubes

¼ teaspoon vanilla

Folic Acid: 🍎🍎
Vitamin B$_{12}$: 🍎🍎🍎
Protein: 🍎🍎
Iron: 🍎
Zinc: 🍎
Calcium: 🍎🍎🍎
Vitamin D: 🍎

1. Cover the dates with water and allow to soak for at least 10 minutes.
2. Discard the soaking water and add the dates and all other ingredients to the blender.
3. Process on medium until smooth, about 1 minute.

Per Serving
Calories: 439 | Fat: 4g | Sodium: 93mg | Fiber: 11g | Protein: 9g

For a Smoother Smoothie

Soaking your dates first will help them process a little quicker and results in a smoother consistency. Place dates in a small bowl and cover with water. Let them sit for about 10 minutes, then drain.

Peanut Butter Granola Wrap

Eating on the go? This wrap has all you need for a healthy breakfast, including whole grains, fresh fruit, and protein. It's the perfect breakfast for someone with a baby bump!

SERVES 1

2 tablespoons peanut butter (or other nut butter)

1 whole-wheat flour tortilla

2 tablespoons granola (or any vegan breakfast cereal)

½ banana, sliced thin

¼ teaspoon cinnamon

1 tablespoon raisins

1 teaspoon agave nectar (optional)

Folic Acid: 🍎

Vitamin B$_{12}$: NA

Protein: 🍎 🍎

Iron: 🍎

Zinc: 🍎 🍎

Calcium: 🍎 🍎

Vitamin D: NA

1. Spread peanut butter down the center of the tortilla and layer granola and banana on top.
2. Sprinkle with cinnamon and raisins and drizzle with agave nectar if desired.
3. Warm in the microwave for 10–15 seconds to slightly melt peanut butter.

Per Serving
Calories: 423 | Fat: 21g | Sodium: 368mg | Fiber: 8g | Protein: 13g

Quick Tofu Breakfast Burrito

Toss in a fresh diced chili if you need something to really wake you up in the morning. There's no reason you can't enjoy these burritos for lunch, either!

SERVES 4

1 (16-ounce) block firm or extra-firm tofu, well pressed

2 tablespoons olive oil

½ cup salsa

½ teaspoon chili powder

Salt and pepper, to taste

4 flour tortillas, warmed

Ketchup or hot sauce, to taste

4 slices vegan cheese

1 avocado, sliced

Folic Acid: 🍎🍎🍎

Vitamin B₁₂: NA

Protein: 🍎🍎🍎

Iron: 🍎🍎

Zinc: 🍎🍎

Calcium: 🍎🍎🍎

Vitamin D: NA

1. Cube or crumble the tofu into 1" chunks. Sauté in olive oil over medium heat for 2–3 minutes.
2. Add salsa and chili powder, and cook for 2–3 more minutes, stirring frequently. Season generously with salt and pepper.
3. Layer each warmed tortilla with ¼ of the tofu and salsa mix and drizzle with ketchup or hot sauce.
4. Add vegan cheese and avocado slices and wrap like a burrito.

Per Serving
Calories: 470 | Fat: 27g | Sodium: 753mg | Fiber: 8g | Protein: 15g

Apple Cinnamon Waffles

For perfect vegan waffles, make sure your waffle iron is hot and very well greased, as vegan waffles tend to be stickier than nonvegan waffles.

SERVES 4

1¼ cups flour

2 teaspoons baking powder

½ teaspoon cinnamon

2 teaspoons sugar

1 cup fortified soymilk

½ cup applesauce

1 teaspoon vanilla

1 tablespoon vegetable oil

Folic Acid: 🍎🍎

Vitamin B$_{12}$: 🍎🍎🍎

Protein: 🍎

Iron: 🍎

Zinc: 🍎

Calcium: 🍎🍎🍎

Vitamin D: 🍎

1. In a large bowl, combine the flour, baking powder, cinnamon, and sugar. Set aside.
2. In a separate bowl, combine soymilk, applesauce, vanilla, and oil.
3. Add the soymilk mixture to the dry ingredients, stirring just until combined; do not overmix.
4. Carefully drop about ¼ cup batter onto preheated waffle iron for each waffle, and cook until done.

Per Serving
Calories: 230 | Fat: 5g | Sodium: 270mg | Fiber: 2g | Protein: 6g

Granola Breakfast Parfait

Sneak some healthy flax meal or wheat germ into your morning meal by adding it to a layered soy yogurt and granola parfait. If you don't have fresh fruit on hand, try adding some dried fruit, such as chopped dried apricots or pineapple. Serve in glass bowls or cups for a nice presentation.

SERVES 2

¼ cup flax meal or wheat germ

2 (6-ounce) containers soy yogurt, any flavor

2 tablespoons maple syrup or agave nectar (optional)

½ cup granola

½ cup sliced fruit

Folic Acid: only present in very small amounts

Vitamin B$_{12}$: 🍎

Protein: 🍎🍎

Iron: 🍎

Zinc: 🍎

Calcium: 🍎🍎🍎

Vitamin D: NA

1. In a small bowl, combine the flax meal or wheat germ, yogurt, and maple syrup.

2. In two serving bowls, place a few spoonfuls of granola, then a layer of soy yogurt. Top with a layer of fresh fruit, and continue layering until ingredients are used up. Serve immediately.

Per Serving
Calories: 354 | Fat: 10g | Sodium: 40mg | Fiber: 8g | Protein: 10g

Maple-Cinnamon Breakfast Quinoa

Quinoa is a filling and healthy breakfast and has more protein than regular oatmeal. This is a deliciously sweet and energizing way to kick off your day.

SERVES 4

1 cup quinoa

2–2½ cups water

1 teaspoon vegan margarine

⅔ cup soymilk

½ teaspoon cinnamon

2 tablespoons maple syrup

2 tablespoons raisins (optional)

2 bananas, sliced (optional)

Folic Acid: 🍎🍎

Vitamin B$_{12}$: 🍎🍎

Protein: 🍎

Iron: 🍎

Zinc: 🍎🍎

Calcium: 🍎

Vitamin D: 🍎

① In a small saucepan, bring the quinoa and water to a boil. Reduce to a simmer and allow to cook, covered, for 15 minutes, until liquid is absorbed.

② Remove from heat and fluff the quinoa with a fork. Cover, and allow to sit for 5 minutes.

③ Stir in the margarine and soymilk, then remaining ingredients.

Per Serving

Calories: 208 | Fat: 4g | Sodium: 39mg | Fiber: 4g | Protein: 7g

No-Sugar Apricot Applesauce

You don't really need to peel the apples if you're short on time, but it only takes about 5 minutes and will give you a smoother sauce. Try adding a touch of nutmeg or pumpkin pie spice for extra flavor.

YIELDS 4 CUPS

6 apples

⅓ cup water

½ cup dried apricots, chopped

4 dates, chopped

Cinnamon, to taste (optional)

Folic Acid: only present in very small amounts

Vitamin B$_{12}$: NA

Protein: 🍎

Iron: 🍎

Zinc: 🍎

Calcium: only present in very small amounts

Vitamin D: NA

1. Peel, core, and chop apples.
2. In a large soup or stockpot, add apples and water and bring to a low boil. Simmer, covered, for 15 minutes, stirring occasionally.
3. Add chopped apricots and dates; simmer for another 10–15 minutes.
4. Mash with a large fork until desired consistency is reached, or allow to cool slightly and purée in a blender until smooth.
5. Sprinkle with cinnamon, to taste.

Per ½ Cup
Calories: 109 | Fat: 0g | Sodium: 1mg | Fiber: 2g | Protein: 1g

Fat-Free Banana Bread

You can add ½ cup chopped walnuts to this simple banana bread, but then, of course, it won't be fat free. If you want a bit of texture without the fat, try adding chopped dates or raisins instead.

YIELDS 1 LOAF

4 ripe bananas

⅓ cup soymilk

⅔ cup sugar

1 teaspoon vanilla

2 cups all-purpose flour

1 teaspoon baking powder

½ teaspoon baking soda

½ teaspoon salt

¾ teaspoon cinnamon

Folic Acid: 🍎🍎

Vitamin B$_{12}$: 🍎

Protein: 🍎

Iron: 🍎

Zinc: 🍎

Calcium: 🍎

Vitamin D: only present in very small amounts

1. Preheat oven to 350°F. Lightly grease a loaf pan.
2. Mix together the bananas, soymilk, sugar, and vanilla until smooth and creamy.
3. In a separate bowl, combine the flour, baking powder, baking soda, and salt.
4. Combine the flour mixture with the banana mixture just until smooth.
5. Spread batter in loaf pan and sprinkle the top with cinnamon. Bake for 55 minutes, or until a toothpick inserted in the middle comes out clean.

Per ⅛ Loaf
Calories: 237 | Fat: 0g | Sodium: 288mg | Fiber: 3g | Protein: 4g

Quick and Easy Vegan Biscuits

Serve these biscuits warm from the oven with apple butter or your favorite jam. These are especially delicious on days when you just don't feel like eating.

YIELDS 12–14 BISCUITS

2 cups flour

1 tablespoon baking powder

½ teaspoon salt

5 tablespoons cold vegan margarine

⅔ cup unsweetened soymilk

Folic Acid: 🍎

Vitamin B$_{12}$: 🍎

Protein: 🍎

Iron: 🍎

Zinc: 🍎

Calcium: 🍎

Vitamin D: only present in very small amounts

1. Preheat oven to 425°F. Lightly grease a baking sheet.
2. Combine flour, baking powder, and salt in a large bowl. Add margarine.
3. Using a fork, mash the margarine with the dry ingredients until crumbly.
4. Add soymilk a few tablespoons at a time; combine just until dough forms. You may need to add a little more or less than ⅔ cup.
5. Knead a few times on a floured surface, then roll out to ¾" thick. Cut into 3" rounds.
6. Bake for 12–14 minutes, or until done.

Per Biscuit
Calories: 125 | Fat: 5g | Sodium: 211mg | Fiber: 1g | Protein: 3g

Vanilla Flax Granola

Making your own granola allows you to create whatever flavors you desire. Add whatever you're craving to the mix!

MAKES 3 CUPS

⅔ cup maple syrup

⅓ cup vegan margarine

1½ teaspoons vanilla

2 cups oats

½ cup flax meal or wheat germ

¾ cup dried fruit, diced small

Folic Acid: only present in very small amounts

Vitamin B$_{12}$: NA

Protein: 🍎

Iron: 🍎

Zinc: 🍎🍎🍎

Calcium: 🍎

Vitamin D: NA

1. Preheat oven to 325°F.
2. Over low heat, melt and whisk together maple syrup, margarine, and vanilla until margarine is melted.
3. Toss together oats, flax meal, and fruit on a large baking tray in a single layer (you may need to use 2 trays).
4. Drizzle maple syrup mixture over oats and fruit; gently toss to combine.
5. Bake for 25–30 minutes, carefully tossing once during cooking. Granola will harden as it cools.

Per ½ Cup
Calories: 368 | Fat: 15g | Sodium: 150mg | Fiber: 7g | Protein: 6g

Morning Cereal Bars

Store-bought breakfast bars are often loaded with artificial sugars, and most homemade recipes require corn syrup. This healthier method makes a sweet and filling snack or breakfast to munch on the run.

YIELDS 14 BARS

3 cups fortified vegan breakfast cereal, any kind

1 cup peanut butter

⅓ cup tahini

1 cup maple syrup

½ teaspoon vanilla

2 cups muesli

½ cup flax meal or wheat germ

½ cup diced dried fruit or raisins

Folic Acid: 🍎🍎

Vitamin B$_{12}$: 🍎🍎🍎

Protein: 🍎🍎

Iron: 🍎🍎

Zinc: 🍎🍎

Calcium: 🍎

Vitamin D: only present in small amounts

1. Lightly grease a baking pan or 2 casserole pans.
2. Place cereal in a sealable bag and crush partially with a rolling pin. If you're using a smaller cereal, you can skip this step. Set aside.
3. Combine peanut butter, tahini, and maple syrup in a large saucepan over low heat, stirring well to combine.
4. Remove from heat and stir in the vanilla, then the cereal, muesli, flax meal or wheat germ, and dried fruit or raisins.
5. Press firmly into greased baking pan and chill until firm, about 45 minutes. Slice into bars.

Per Bar
Calories: 314 | Fat: 15g | Sodium: 166mg | Fiber: 5g | Protein: 9g

Sweet Potato Apple Latkes

Serve these latkes topped with No-Sugar Apricot Applesauce (see recipe in this chapter) or nondairy sour cream.

YIELDS 1 DOZEN LATKES

3 large sweet potatoes, peeled and grated

1 apple, grated

1 small yellow onion, grated

Egg replacer for 2 eggs

3 tablespoons flour

1 teaspoon baking powder

½ teaspoon cinnamon

½ teaspoon nutmeg

½ teaspoon salt

Oil for frying

Folic Acid: only present in very small amounts

Vitamin B$_{12}$: NA

Protein: 🍎

Iron: only present in very small amounts

Zinc: 🍎

Calcium: 🍎

Vitamin D: NA

1. Using a cloth or paper towel, gently squeeze out excess moisture from potatoes and apples; combine with onions in a large bowl.
2. Mix together remaining ingredients except oil; combine with potato mixture.
3. In a skillet or frying pan, heat a few tablespoons of oil. Drop potato mixture in the hot oil a scant ¼ cup at a time. Use a spatula to flatten, forming a pancake. Cook for 3–4 minutes on each side, until lightly crisped.

Per Latke
Calories: 89 | Fat: 4g | Sodium: 162mg | Fiber: 2g | Protein: 1g

Super Green Quiche

Get your greens in before noon with this veggie quiche.

SERVES 4

1 (10-ounce) package frozen chopped spinach, thawed and drained

½ cup broccoli, diced small

1 (16-ounce) block firm or extra-firm tofu

1 tablespoon soy sauce

¼ cup soymilk

1 teaspoon prepared mustard

2 tablespoons nutritional yeast

½ teaspoon garlic powder

1 teaspoon parsley

½ teaspoon rosemary

¾ teaspoon salt

¼ teaspoon pepper

Prepared vegan crust

Folic Acid: 🍎🍎🍎

Vitamin B$_{12}$: 🍎🍎🍎

Protein: 🍎🍎🍎

Iron: 🍎🍎

Zinc: 🍎🍎🍎

Calcium: 🍎🍎🍎

Vitamin D: only present in small amounts

1. Preheat oven to 350°F.
2. Steam the spinach and broccoli until just lightly cooked, then set aside to cool. Press as much moisture as possible out of the spinach.
3. In a blender or food processor, combine the tofu with the remaining ingredients except crust until well mixed. Mix in the spinach and broccoli by hand until combined.
4. Spread mixture evenly in pie crust.
5. Bake for 35–40 minutes, or until firm. Allow to cool for at least 10 minutes before serving. Quiche will firm up a bit more as it cools.

Per Serving
Calories: 403 | Fat: 20g | Sodium: 1,560mg | Fiber: 7g | Protein: 17g

Vegan Pancakes

A touch of sugar and hint of sweet banana flavor make this pancake recipe sparkle.

YIELDS 1 DOZEN PANCAKES

1 cup flour

1 tablespoon sugar

1¾ teaspoons baking powder

¼ teaspoon salt

½ banana

1 teaspoon vanilla

1 cup soymilk

Folic Acid: 🍎

Vitamin B$_{12}$: 🍎

Protein: 🍎

Iron: 🍎

Zinc: only present in very small amounts

Calcium: 🍎

Vitamin D: only present in very small amounts

1. In a large bowl, mix together flour, sugar, baking powder, and salt.
2. In a separate small bowl, mash banana with a fork. Add vanilla; whisk until smooth and fluffy. Add soymilk; stir to combine well.
3. Add wet mixture to dry ingredients; stir.
4. Heat a lightly greased griddle or large frying pan over medium heat. Drop batter about 3 tablespoons at a time and heat until bubbles appear on surface, about 2–3 minutes. Flip and cook other side until lightly golden brown, another 1–2 minutes.

Per Pancake
Calories: 56 | Fat: 0g | Sodium: 128mg | Fiber: 0g | Protein: 2g

Baked "Sausage" and Mushroom Frittata

Baked tofu frittatas are an easy brunch or weekend breakfast. Once you've got the technique down, it's easy to adjust the ingredients to your liking. With tofu and mock meat, this one packs a super protein punch!

SERVES 4

½ yellow onion, diced

3 cloves garlic, minced

½ cup sliced mushrooms

1 (12-ounce) package vegetarian sausage substitute or vegetarian "beef" crumbles

2 tablespoons olive oil

¾ teaspoon salt, or to taste

¼ teaspoon black pepper

1 (16-ounce) block firm or extra-firm tofu

1 (12-ounce) block silken tofu

1 tablespoon soy sauce

2 tablespoons nutritional yeast

¼ teaspoon turmeric (optional)

1 tomato, sliced thin (optional)

Folic Acid: 🍎🍎🍎

Vitamin B₁₂: 🍎🍎🍎

Protein: 🍎🍎🍎

Iron: 🍎🍎

Zinc: 🍎🍎🍎

Calcium: 🍎🍎🍎

Vitamin D: only present in small amounts

1. Preheat oven to 325°F and lightly grease a glass pie pan.
2. In a large skillet, heat onion, garlic, mushrooms, and vegetarian sausage in olive oil until sausage is browned and mushrooms are soft, about 3–4 minutes. Season with salt and pepper and set aside.
3. Combine firm tofu, silken tofu, soy sauce, nutritional yeast, and turmeric in a blender; process until mixed. Combine tofu mixture with sausage mixture; spread into pan. Layer slices of tomato on top (optional).
4. Bake in oven for about 45 minutes, or until firm. Allow to cool for 5–10 minutes before serving, as frittata will set as it cools.

Per Serving
Calories: 301 | Fat: 17g | Sodium: 1,037mg | Fiber: 4g | Protein: 25g

Chili Masala Tofu Scramble

Tofu scramble is an easy and versatile vegan breakfast. This version adds chili and curry for continental flavor. Toss in whatever veggies you have on hand—tomatoes, spinach, or diced broccoli would work well.

SERVES 4

1 (16-ounce) block firm or extra-firm tofu, pressed

1 small onion, diced

2 cloves garlic, minced

2 tablespoons olive oil

1 small red chili pepper, minced

1 green bell pepper, chopped

¾ cup sliced mushrooms

1 tablespoon soy sauce

1 teaspoon curry powder

½ teaspoon cumin

¼ teaspoon turmeric

1 teaspoon nutritional yeast (optional)

Folic Acid: 🍎

Vitamin B$_{12}$: NA

Protein: 🍎🍎

Iron: 🍎

Zinc: 🍎

Calcium: 🍎🍎

Vitamin D: only present in very small amounts

1. Cut pressed tofu into 1" cubes or crumble into medium-small pieces.
2. Sauté onion and garlic in olive oil until onions are soft, about 1–2 minutes.
3. Add tofu, chili pepper, bell pepper, and mushrooms, stirring well to combine.
4. Add remaining ingredients, except nutritional yeast, and combine well. Cook until tofu is lightly browned, about 6–8 minutes.
5. Remove from heat and stir in nutritional yeast if desired.

Per Serving
Calories: 144 | Fat: 10g | Sodium: 240mg | Fiber: 2g | Protein: 8g

The Next Day

Leftover tofu scramble makes an excellent lunch, or wrap leftovers in a warmed flour tortilla to make breakfast-style burritos, perhaps with some salsa or beans. Why isn't it called scrambled tofu instead of tofu scramble if it's a substitute for scrambled eggs? This is one of the great conundrums of veganism.

Easy Vegan French Toast

For a leisurely weekend breakfast, try golden-fried French toast topped with a fruit compote or some agave nectar or maple syrup.

SERVES 4

2 bananas

½ cup soymilk

1 tablespoon orange juice

1 tablespoon maple syrup

¾ teaspoon vanilla

1 tablespoon flour

1 teaspoon cinnamon

½ teaspoon nutmeg

Oil or vegan margarine, for frying

12 thick slices bread

Folic Acid: 🍏 🍏

Vitamin B₁₂: 🍏 🍏

Protein: 🍏 🍏

Iron: 🍏 🍏

Zinc: 🍏

Calcium: 🍏 🍏

Vitamin D: 🍏

1. Using a blender or mixer, mix together the bananas, soymilk, orange juice, maple syrup, and vanilla until smooth and creamy.
2. Whisk in flour, cinnamon, and nutmeg; pour into a pie plate or shallow pan.
3. In a large skillet, heat 1–2 tablespoons of vegan margarine or oil.
4. Dip or spoon mixture over each bread slice on both sides and fry in hot oil until lightly golden brown on both sides, about 2–3 minutes.

Per Serving
Calories: 391 | Fat: 11g | Sodium: 629mg | Fiber: 4g | Protein: 9g

The Perfect Vegan French Toast

Creating an eggless French toast is a true art. Is your French toast too soggy or too dry? Thickly sliced bread lightly toasted will be more absorbent. Too mushy, or the mixture doesn't want to stick? Try spooning it onto your bread, rather than dipping.

Whole-Wheat Blueberry Muffins

Because these muffins have very little fat, they'll want to stick to the papers or the muffin tin. Letting them cool before removing them will help prevent this, as will greasing your muffin tin well.

YIELDS ABOUT 1½ DOZEN MUFFINS

2 cups whole-wheat flour

1 cup all-purpose flour

1¼ cups sugar

1 tablespoon baking powder

1 teaspoon salt

1½ cups fortified soymilk

½ cup applesauce

½ teaspoon vanilla

2 cups blueberries

Folic Acid: 🍎

Vitamin B$_{12}$: 🍎

Protein: 🍎

Iron: 🍎

Zinc: 🍎

Calcium: 🍎

Vitamin D: only present in very small amounts

1. Preheat oven to 400°F. Line or grease muffin tins.
2. In a large bowl, combine the flours, sugar, baking powder, and salt. Set aside.
3. In a separate small bowl, whisk together the soymilk, applesauce, and vanilla until well mixed.
4. Combine the wet ingredients with the dry ingredients; stir just until mixed. Gently fold in ½ of the blueberries.
5. Spoon batter into muffin tins, filling each tin about ⅔ full. Sprinkle remaining blueberries on top of muffins.
6. Bake for 20–25 minutes, or until lightly golden brown on top.

Per Muffin
Calories: 147 | Fat: 1g | Sodium: 220mg | Fiber: 2g | Protein: 3g

Making Vegan Muffins

Got a favorite muffin recipe? Try making it vegan! Use a commercial egg replacer in place of the eggs, and substitute a vegan soy margarine and soymilk for the butter and milk. Voilà!

Homemade Nut Milk

Homemade nut milk is delicious in breakfast cereal or oatmeal, smoothies, or to use in baking. If you don't have a sieve or cheesecloth, you can still enjoy this recipe, but it will be a bit grainy.

YIELDS 4 CUPS

1 cup raw almonds or cashews

Water for soaking

4 cups water

½ teaspoon salt

½ teaspoon vanilla

1 teaspoon sugar (optional)

Folic Acid: 🍎

Vitamin B$_{12}$: NA

Protein: 🍎🍎

Iron: 🍎

Zinc: 🍎

Calcium: 🍎🍎

Vitamin D: NA

1. In a large bowl, cover nuts with plenty of water and allow to soak for at least 1 hour, or overnight. Drain.
2. Blend together soaked nuts with 4 cups water and purée on high until smooth.
3. Strain through a cheesecloth or sieve.
4. Stir in salt, vanilla, and sugar, and adjust to taste.

Per Cup
Calories: 189 | Fat: 16g | Sodium: 296mg | Fiber: 0g | Protein: 8g

Does It Taste Different Than What You Expected?

If you read the label of most nondairy milks, you'll find them loaded with sugar! The first few times you make a homemade batch, you may need to add extra sugar to replicate the store-bought taste. Or, try using a healthier sweetener, such as maple syrup or agave nectar.

Vegan Crepes

Crepes make a lovely brunch or even dessert, depending on what you fill them with! During your pregnancy, fill them up with whatever you're craving and enjoy!

SERVES 4

1 cup flour

¾ cup soymilk

¼ cup water

2 teaspoons sugar

1 teaspoon vanilla

¼ cup vegan margarine, melted

¼ teaspoon salt

Folic Acid: 🍎

Vitamin B$_{12}$: 🍎🍎🍎

Protein: 🍎

Iron: 🍎

Zinc: 🍎

Calcium: 🍎

Vitamin D: 🍎

① Whisk together all ingredients. Chill for at least 1 hour. Remove from fridge and remix.

② Lightly grease a nonstick pan and heat over medium-high heat.

③ Place about ¼ cup batter in pan and swirl to coat. Cook for just a minute, until set, then carefully flip, using a spatula or even your hands. Heat for just 1 more minute, then transfer to a plate.

Per Serving
Calories: 221 | Fat: 12g | Sodium: 336mg | Fiber: 1g | Protein: 4g

It's All in the Wrist

Don't worry if the first one or two turn out less than perfect; it always seems to happen. As you master the swirl technique, you'll soon be churning out perfect crepes every time. If you've never tried, you may want to make a double batch so you can practice. Be sure to use a nonstick pan!

Tofu Florentine

Satisfy your comfort food cravings with this "eggy" tofu and spinach mixture drowning in a creamy Quick Hollandaise Sauce (see recipe in this chapter) on toast.

SERVES 2

1 (16-ounce) block firm or extra-firm tofu, well pressed

2 tablespoons flour

1 teaspoon nutritional yeast

1 teaspoon garlic powder

2 tablespoons canola or safflower oil

1 (10-ounce) box frozen spinach, thawed and drained

½ cup Quick Hollandaise Sauce (see recipe in this chapter)

2 slices bread, lightly toasted (or English muffins or bagels)

Folic Acid: 🍎🍎🍎
Vitamin B$_{12}$: 🍎🍎
Protein: 🍎🍎🍎
Iron: 🍎🍎🍎
Zinc: 🍎🍎🍎
Calcium: 🍎🍎🍎
Vitamin D: NA

1. Slice tofu into ½"-thick slabs.
2. In a small bowl, combine the flour, nutritional yeast, and garlic powder. Dredge tofu in this mixture, then fry in oil for 2–3 minutes on each side until lightly browned.
3. Reduce heat and add spinach and 2 tablespoons of hollandaise sauce, gently coating tofu. Cook for just a minute or two over low heat until spinach is heated through.
4. Stack spinach and 2 strips of tofu mixture on each piece of toasted bread and cover with remaining sauce.

Per Serving
Calories: 436 | Fat: 26g | Sodium: 412mg | Fiber: 7g | Protein: 23g

Benedict vs. Florentine

For a variation on this classic brunch recipe, skip the spinach and add a layer of lightly browned store-bought vegan bacon for Eggs Benedict instead of Florentine.

Quick Hollandaise Sauce

A classic Hollandaise sauce is made from raw eggs, but this vegan cheater's version uses prepared vegan mayonnaise with a bit of turmeric for a yellow hue. Pour over steamed asparagus, artichokes, or cauliflower for an easy side dish, or make Tofu Florentine (see recipe in this chapter) or "eggs" Benedict.

YIELDS ½ CUP

⅓ cup vegan mayonnaise

¼ cup lemon juice

3 tablespoons unsweetened soymilk

1½ tablespoons Dijon mustard

¼ teaspoon turmeric

1 tablespoon nutritional yeast (optional)

½ teaspoon salt

¼ teaspoon black pepper

¼ teaspoon hot sauce, or to taste (optional)

Folic Acid: only present in very small amounts

Vitamin B$_{12}$: 🍎

Protein: only present in very small amounts

Iron: only present in very small amounts

Zinc: NA

Calcium: only present in very small amounts

Vitamin D: NA

- Whisk together all ingredients and heat over low heat before serving. Adjust seasonings to taste.

Per Tablespoon
Calories: 66 | Fat: 6g | Sodium: 163mg | Fiber: 0g | Protein: 0g

Potato Poblano Breakfast Burritos

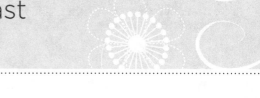

With or without the optional ingredients, this is a filling breakfast. Plan on two servings without the vegetarian ground beef, or stretch it to three servings with the mock meat.

SERVES 2

2 tablespoons olive oil

2 small potatoes, diced small

2 poblano or Anaheim chilies, diced

1 teaspoon chili powder

Salt and pepper to taste

1 tomato, diced

⅔ cup vegetarian ground beef or sausage substitute (optional)

2–3 flour tortillas, warmed

Grated vegan cheese (optional)

Ketchup or hot sauce (optional)

Folic Acid: 🌶🌶

Vitamin B$_{12}$: NA

Protein: 🌶🌶

Iron: 🌶🌶

Zinc: 🌶

Calcium: 🌶🌶

Vitamin D: NA

1. Heat olive oil in a pan and add potatoes and chilies, sautéing until potatoes are almost soft, about 6–7 minutes.
2. Add chili powder, salt and pepper, tomato, and meat substitute, and stir well to combine.
3. Continue cooking until potatoes and tomatoes are soft and meat substitute is cooked, another 4–5 minutes.
4. Wrap in warmed flour tortillas with vegan cheese and ketchup or a bit of hot sauce, if desired.

Per Serving
Calories: 353 | Fat: 9g | Sodium: 322mg | Fiber: 8g | Protein: 9g

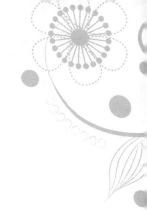

CHAPTER 4

Appetizers

Black Bean Guacamole

Sneaking some extra fiber and protein into a traditional Mexican guacamole makes this dip a more nutritious snack or appetizer.

YIELDS 2 CUPS

1 (15-ounce) can black beans, drained and rinsed

3 avocados, pitted

1 tablespoon lime juice

3 scallions, chopped

1 large tomato, diced

2 cloves garlic, minced

½ teaspoon chili powder

¼ teaspoon salt, or to taste

1 tablespoon chopped fresh cilantro

Folic Acid: 🍎🍎

Vitamin B$_{12}$: NA

Protein: 🍎

Iron: 🍎

Zinc: 🍎

Calcium: 🍎

Vitamin D: NA

1. In a medium-sized bowl, using a fork or a potato masher, mash the beans just until they are halfway mashed, leaving some texture.
2. Add the remaining ingredients; mash together until mixed.
3. Adjust seasonings to taste.
4. Allow to sit for at least 10 minutes before serving to allow the flavors to set.
5. Gently mix again just before serving.

Per ¼ Cup
Calories: 198 | Fat: 11g | Sodium: 206mg | Fiber: 10g | Protein: 7g

Easy Vegan Pizza Bagels

Need a quick lunch, after-work, or in-the-middle-of-the-night snack? Pizza bagels to the rescue! For a real treat, shop for vegetarian "pepperoni" slices to top it off!

SERVES 4

⅓ cup vegan pizza sauce or tomato sauce

½ teaspoon garlic powder

¼ teaspoon salt, or to taste

½ teaspoon basil

½ teaspoon oregano

4 vegan bagels, sliced in half

8 slices vegan cheese or 1 cup grated vegan cheese

¼ cup sliced mushrooms (optional)

¼ cup sliced black olives

Folic Acid: 🍎🍎

Vitamin B₁₂: 🍎🍎

Protein: 🍎🍎

Iron: 🍎🍎

Zinc: 🍎🍎

Calcium: 🍎🍎🍎

Vitamin D: NA

1. Preheat oven to 325°F.
2. Combine pizza sauce, garlic powder, salt, basil, and oregano.
3. Spread sauce over each bagel half; top with cheese, mushrooms, olives, or any other toppings.
4. Heat in oven for 8–10 minutes, or until cheese is melted.

Per Serving
Calories: 308 | Fat: 9g | Sodium: 900mg | Fiber: 2g | Protein: 13g

Eggplant Baba Ghanoush

Whip up a batch of Eggplant Baba Ghanoush, Roasted Red Pepper Hummus, and some Vegan Tzatziki (see recipes in this chapter) and make a Mediterranean appetizer spread. Don't forget some vegan pita bread to dip into your baba.

YIELDS 1½ CUPS

2 medium eggplants

3 tablespoons olive oil

2 tablespoons lemon juice

¼ cup tahini

3 cloves garlic, minced

½ teaspoon cumin

½ teaspoon chili powder (optional)

¼ teaspoon salt, or to taste

1 tablespoon chopped fresh parsley

Folic Acid: 🍎

Vitamin B$_{12}$: NA

Protein: 🍎

Iron: 🍎

Zinc: 🍎

Calcium: 🍎

Vitamin D: NA

1. Preheat oven to 400°F.
2. Slice eggplants in half; prick several times with a fork.
3. Place on a baking sheet; drizzle with 1 tablespoon olive oil. Bake for 30 minutes, or until soft. Allow to cool slightly.
4. Remove inner flesh; place in a bowl.
5. Using a large fork or potato masher, mash eggplant together with remaining ingredients until almost smooth.
6. Adjust seasonings, to taste.

Per ¼ Cup
Calories: 161 | Fat: 13g | Sodium: 113mg | Fiber: 6g | Protein: 3g

Green and Black Olive Tapenade

This olive tapenade can be used as a spread or dip for baguettes or crackers. If you don't have a food processor, you could also mash the ingredients together with a mortar and pestle or a large fork.

YIELDS 1 CUP

½ cup pitted green olives

¾ cup pitted black olives

2 cloves garlic

1 tablespoon capers (optional)

2 tablespoons lemon juice

2 tablespoons olive oil

¼ teaspoon oregano

¼ teaspoon black pepper

Folic Acid: only present in very small amounts

Vitamin B$_{12}$: NA

Protein: only present in very small amounts

Iron: only present in very small amounts

Zinc: NA

Calcium: only present in very small amounts

Vitamin D: NA

● Process all ingredients in a food processor until almost smooth.

Per Tablespoon
Calories: 29 | Fat: 3g | Sodium: 116mg | Fiber: 0g | Protein: 0g

Hot Artichoke Spinach Dip

Serve this creamy dip hot with some baguette slices, crackers, pita bread, or sliced bell peppers and jicama. If you want to get fancy, you can carve out a bread bowl for an edible serving dish.

SERVES 8

1 (12-ounce) package frozen spinach, thawed

1 (14-ounce) can artichoke hearts, drained

¼ cup vegan margarine

¼ cup flour

2 cups fortified soymilk

½ cup nutritional yeast

1 teaspoon garlic powder

1½ teaspoons onion powder

¼ teaspoon salt, or to taste

Folic Acid: 🍎🍎🍎

Vitamin B$_{12}$: 🍎🍎🍎

Protein: 🍎

Iron: 🍎

Zinc: 🍎🍎

Calcium: 🍎🍎

Vitamin D: 🍎

① Preheat oven to 350°F. Purée spinach and artichokes together until almost smooth; set aside.

② In a small saucepan, melt the margarine over low heat. Slowly whisk in flour, 1 tablespoon at a time, stirring constantly to avoid lumps, until thick, about 1–3 minutes.

③ Remove from heat and add spinach and artichoke mixture; stir to combine. Add remaining ingredients.

④ Transfer to an ovenproof casserole dish or bowl; bake for 20 minutes. Serve hot.

Per Serving
Calories: 134 | Fat: 7g | Sodium: 378mg | Fiber: 4g | Protein: 6g

Mango Citrus Salsa

Salsa has a variety of uses, and this recipe adds color and variety to your usual chips and dip or Mexican dishes.

YIELDS 2 CUPS

1 mango, peeled and chopped

2 tangerines, peeled and chopped

½ red bell pepper, chopped

½ red onion, minced

3 cloves garlic, minced

½ jalapeño pepper, minced

2 tablespoons lime juice

½ teaspoon salt, or to taste

¼ teaspoon black pepper

3 tablespoons chopped fresh cilantro

Folic Acid: 🍎

Vitamin B$_{12}$: NA

Protein: 🍎

Iron: only present in very small amounts

Zinc: only present in very small amounts

Calcium: only present in very small amounts

Vitamin D: NA

① Gently toss together all ingredients.

② Allow to sit for at least 15 minutes before serving to allow flavors to mingle.

Per ¼ Cup
Calories: 37 | Fat: 0g | Sodium: 147mg | Fiber: 1g | Protein: 1g

Roasted Cashew and Spicy Basil Pesto

The combination of spicy purple Thai basil (or holy basil instead of Italian sweet basil) and the bite of the garlic creates an electrifying vegan pesto.

SERVES 3

4 cloves garlic

1 cup Thai basil or holy basil, packed

⅔ cup roasted cashews

½ cup nutritional yeast

¾ teaspoon salt, or to taste

½ teaspoon black pepper

⅓–½ cup olive oil

Folic Acid: 🍎🍎🍎

Vitamin B₁₂: 🍎🍎🍎 Includes 100% of the DRI

Protein: 🍎🍎

Iron: 🍎🍎

Zinc: 🍎🍎🍎

Calcium: 🍎

Vitamin D: NA

1. In a blender or food processor, process all ingredients except olive oil just until coarse and combined.
2. Slowly incorporate olive oil until desired consistency is reached.

Per Serving
Calories: 435 | Fat: 38g | Sodium: 779mg | Fiber: 4g | Protein: 10g

Roasted Red Pepper Hummus

You'll rarely meet a vegan who doesn't love hummus in one form or another. As a veggie dip or sandwich spread, hummus is always a favorite. Up the garlic in this recipe, if that's your thing, and don't be ashamed to lick the spoons or spatula.

YIELDS 1½ CUPS

1 (15-ounce) can chickpeas, drained and rinsed

⅓ cup tahini

⅔ cup chopped roasted red peppers

3 tablespoons lemon juice

2 tablespoons olive oil

2 cloves garlic

½ teaspoon cumin

⅓ teaspoon salt, or to taste

¼ teaspoon cayenne pepper (optional)

Folic Acid: 🍎🍎

Vitamin B$_{12}$: NA

Protein: 🍎

Iron: 🍎

Zinc: 🍎🍎

Calcium: 🍎

Vitamin D: NA

● In a blender or food processor, process all ingredients until smooth, scraping the sides down as needed.

Per ¼ Cup
Calories: 215 | Fat: 13g | Sodium: 441mg | Fiber: 4g | Protein: 6g

Tropical Cashew Nut Butter

You can make a homemade cashew nut butter with any kind of oil, so feel free to substitute using whatever you have on hand. But you're in for a real treat when you use coconut oil in this recipe!

YIELDS ¾ CUP

2 cups roasted cashews

½ teaspoon sugar (optional)

¼ teaspoon salt (optional)

3–4 tablespoons coconut oil or other vegetable oil

Folic Acid: 🍎

Vitamin B$_{12}$: NA

Protein: 🍎

Iron: 🍎

Zinc: 🍎🍎🍎

Calcium: 🍎

Vitamin D: NA

1. In a food processor on high speed, process the cashews, sugar, and salt until finely ground. Continue processing until cashews form a thick paste.
2. Slowly add coconut oil until smooth and creamy, scraping down sides and adding a little more oil as needed.

Per 2 Tablespoons
Calories: 320 | Fat: 28g | Sodium: 7mg | Fiber: 1g | Protein: 7g

Fresh Basil Bruschetta with Balsamic Reduction

Your guests will be so delighted by the rich flavors of the balsamic reduction sauce that they won't even notice that the cheese is missing from this vegan bruschetta. Use a fresh artisan bread, if you can, for extra flavor.

SERVES 4

8–10 slices vegan French bread

¾ cup balsamic vinegar

1 tablespoon sugar

2 large tomatoes, diced small

3 cloves garlic, minced

2 tablespoons olive oil

¼ cup chopped fresh basil

Salt and pepper, to taste

Folic Acid: 🍎🍎

Vitamin B$_{12}$: NA

Protein: 🍎🍎

Iron: 🍎🍎

Zinc: 🍎

Calcium: 🍎

Vitamin D: NA

1. Toast bread in toaster or for 5 minutes in the oven at 350°F.
2. In a small saucepan, whisk together the balsamic vinegar and sugar. Bring to a boil; reduce to a slow simmer. Allow to cook for 6–8 minutes, until almost thickened. Remove from heat.
3. In a large bowl, combine the tomatoes, garlic, olive oil, basil, salt, and pepper; gently toss with balsamic sauce.
4. Spoon tomato and balsamic mixture over bread slices; serve immediately.

Per Serving
Calories: 321 | Fat: 8g | Sodium: 434mg | Fiber: 3g | Protein: 9g

Mushroom Fondue

Nutritional yeast lends a rich flavor to this fun party fondue. If you don't have a fondue pot, you can mix the ingredients over low heat and serve hot. Don't forget plenty of dippers—vegan French bread, mushrooms, or lightly cooked baby potatoes would work well.

SERVES 4

2 tablespoons vegan margarine

2 cups sliced mushrooms

½ cup unflavored soymilk or soy creamer

1 teaspoon onion powder

½ teaspoon garlic powder

½ teaspoon celery salt

2 tablespoons flour

3 tablespoons nutritional yeast

Folic Acid: 🍎🍎🍎

Vitamin B$_{12}$: 🍎🍎🍎

Protein: 🍎

Iron: 🍎

Zinc: 🍎

Calcium: 🍎

Vitamin D: 🍎

1. Melt the margarine over low heat; add mushrooms. Allow to cook for 5 minutes, then add soymilk, onion powder, garlic powder, and celery salt. Cook for 8–10 minutes, until mushrooms are soft.
2. Allow mixture to cool slightly; purée in a blender.
3. Place puréed mushrooms in a fondue pot.
4. Over medium heat, whisk in flour; heat until thickened, about 2–4 minutes.
5. Stir in nutritional yeast; serve immediately.

Per Serving
Calories: 99 | Fat: 6g | Sodium: 163mg | Fiber: 1g | Protein: 4g

Vegan Cheese Ball

Use this recipe to make one impressive-looking large cheese ball, a cheese log, or individual bite-sized servings for a baby shower or the holidays. Everyone will be asking you for the recipe!

MAKES 1 LARGE CHEESE BALL OR 12–14 BITE-SIZED CHEESE BALLS

1 (10-ounce) block vegan nacho or Cheddar cheese, at room temperature

1 (8-ounce) container vegan cream cheese, at room temperature

1 teaspoon garlic powder

½ teaspoon hot sauce

¼ teaspoon salt, or to taste

1 teaspoon paprika

¼ cup nuts, finely chopped

Folic Acid: only present in very small amounts

Vitamin B$_{12}$: NA

Protein: 🥕

Iron: 🥕

Zinc: only present in very small amounts

Calcium: 🥕

Vitamin D: NA

1. Grate cheese into a large bowl, or process in a food processor until finely minced. Using a large fork, mash the cheese together with the cream cheese, garlic powder, hot sauce, and salt until well mixed. (You may need to use your hands for this.)
2. Chill until firm, at least 1 hour; shape into ball or log, pressing firmly.
3. Sprinkle with paprika; carefully roll in nuts. Serve with crackers.

Per Bite-Sized Cheese Ball
Calories: 132 | Fat: 10g | Sodium: 285mg | Fiber: 2g | Protein: 2g

Vegan Tzatziki

Use a vegan soy yogurt to make this classic Greek dip, which is best served very cold. A nondairy sour cream may be used instead of the soy yogurt, if you prefer.

YIELDS 1½ CUPS

1½ cups vegan soy yogurt, plain or lemon flavored

1 tablespoon olive oil

1 tablespoon lemon juice

4 cloves garlic, minced

2 cucumbers, grated or chopped fine

1 tablespoon chopped fresh mint or fresh dill

Folic Acid: only present in very small amounts

Vitamin B$_{12}$: NA

Protein: 🍏

Iron: only present in very small amounts

Zinc: 🍏

Calcium: 🍏

Vitamin D: 🍏

1. Whisk together yogurt, olive oil, and lemon juice until well combined.
2. Combine with remaining ingredients.
3. Chill for at least 1 hour before serving to allow flavors to mingle. Serve cold.

Per ¼ Cup
Calories: 76 | Fat: 3g | Sodium: 10mg | Fiber: 1g | Protein: 2g

Nacho "Cheese" Dip

Peanut butter in cheese sauce? No, that's not a typo! Just a touch of peanut butter creates a creamy and nutty layer of flavor to this sauce, and helps it to thicken nicely. Use this sauce to dress plain steamed veggies or make homemade nachos.

YIELDS ABOUT 1 CUP

3 tablespoons vegan margarine

1 cup unsweetened soymilk

¾ teaspoon garlic powder

½ teaspoon salt, or to taste

½ teaspoon onion powder

1 tablespoon peanut butter

¼ cup flour

¼ cup nutritional yeast

¾ cup salsa

2 tablespoons chopped canned jalapeño peppers (optional)

Folic Acid: 🍎🍎🍎
Vitamin B$_{12}$: 🍎🍎🍎
Protein: 🍎
Iron: 🍎
Zinc: 🍎🍎
Calcium: 🍎
Vitamin D: NA

1. In a pan over low heat, heat margarine and soymilk.
2. Add garlic powder, salt, and onion powder; stir to combine.
3. Add peanut butter; stir until melted.
4. Whisk in flour, 1 tablespoon at a time, until smooth. Heat until thickened, about 5–6 minutes.
5. Stir in nutritional yeast, salsa, and jalapeño peppers.
6. Allow to cool slightly before serving, as cheese sauce will thicken as it cools.

Per ¼ Cup
Calories: 184 | Fat: 12g | Sodium: 725mg | Fiber: 3g | Protein: 6g

Avocado and Shiitake Pot Stickers

Once you try these California-fusion pot stickers, you'll wish you had made a double batch! These little dumplings don't need to be enhanced with a complex dipping sauce, so serve them plain or with soy sauce.

YIELDS 12–15 POT STICKERS

1 avocado, diced small

½ cup shiitake mushrooms, diced

½ (6-ounce) block silken tofu, crumbled

1 clove garlic, minced

2 teaspoons balsamic vinegar

1 teaspoon soy sauce

12–15 vegan dumpling wrappers

Water for steaming or oil for pan frying

Folic Acid: 🍎

Vitamin B₁₂: NA

Protein: 🍎🍎

Iron: 🍎

Zinc: 🍎

Calcium: only present in very small amounts

Vitamin D: NA

① In a small bowl, gently mash together all ingredients except wrappers, just until mixed and crumbly.

② Place about 1½ teaspoons of the filling in the middle of each wrapper. Fold in half and pinch closed, forming little pleats. You may want to dip your fingertips in water to help the dumplings stay sealed, if needed.

③ *To pan fry:* Heat a thin layer of oil in a large skillet. Carefully add dumplings and cook for just 1 minute. Add about ½ cup water; cover, and cook for 3–4 minutes.

④ *To steam:* Carefully place a layer of dumplings in a steamer, making sure the dumplings don't touch. Place steamer above boiling water; allow to cook, covered, for 3–4 minutes.

Per 2 Pot Stickers (Steamed)
Calories: 304 | Fat: 6g | Sodium: 356mg | Fiber: 4g | Protein: 9g

Whether Steamed or Fried ...

In dumpling houses across East Asia, dumplings are served with a little bowl of freshly grated ginger, and diners create a simple dipping sauce from the various condiments on the table. To try it, pour some rice vinegar and a touch of soy sauce over a bit of ginger and add hot chili oil to taste.

Homemade Tahini

If you're serving this as a Middle Eastern dip or spread, use the paprika for extra flavor, but leave it out if your tahini will be the basis for a salad dressing or a noodle dish.

YIELDS 1 CUP

2 cups sesame seeds

½ cup olive oil

½ teaspoon paprika (optional)

Folic Acid: 🍎

Vitamin B₁₂: NA

Protein: 🍎

Iron: 🍎

Zinc: 🍎 🍎

Calcium: 🍎 🍎

Vitamin D: NA

1. Heat oven to 350°F. Once oven is hot, spread sesame seeds in a thin layer on a baking sheet and toast for 5 minutes in the oven, shaking the sheet once to mix.

2. Allow sesame seeds to cool, then process with oil in a food processor or blender until thick and creamy. You may need a little more or less than ½ cup oil. Garnish with paprika, if desired. Tahini will keep for up to one month in the refrigerator in a tightly sealed container, or store your tahini in the freezer and thaw before using.

Per Tablespoon
Calories: 163 | Fat: 16g | Sodium: 2mg | Fiber: 2g | Protein: 3g

Fresh Mint Spring Rolls

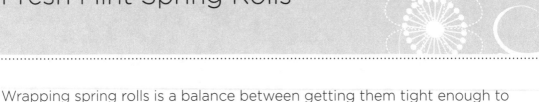

Wrapping spring rolls is a balance between getting them tight enough to hold together, but not so tight that the thin wrappers break! It's like riding a bike: once you've got it, you've got it, and then spring rolls can be very quick and fun to make.

SERVES 4

1 (3-ounce) package clear bean thread noodles

1 cup hot water

1 tablespoon soy sauce

½ teaspoon powdered ginger

1 teaspoon sesame oil

¼ cup diced shiitake mushrooms

1 carrot, grated

10–12 spring roll wrappers

Warm water

½ head green leaf lettuce, chopped

1 cucumber, sliced thin

1 bunch fresh mint

Folic Acid: 🍎

Vitamin B$_{12}$: NA

Protein: 🍎

Iron: 🍎

Zinc: 🍎

Calcium: 🍎

Vitamin D: NA

1. Break noodles in half to make smaller pieces, then submerge in 1 cup hot water until soft, about 6–7 minutes. Drain.
2. In a large bowl, toss together the hot noodles with the soy sauce, ginger, sesame oil, mushrooms, and carrots, tossing well to combine.
3. In a large shallow pan, carefully submerge spring roll wrappers, one at a time, in warm water until just barely soft. Remove from water and place a bit of lettuce in the center of the wrapper. Add about 2 tablespoons of noodle mixture, a few slices of cucumber, and place 2–3 mint leaves on top.
4. Fold the bottom of the wrapper over the filling, fold in each side, then roll.

Per Serving
Calories: 216 | Fat: 1g | Sodium: 262mg | Fiber: 2g | Protein: 4g

Easy Asian Dipping Sauce

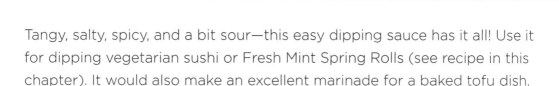

Tangy, salty, spicy, and a bit sour—this easy dipping sauce has it all! Use it for dipping vegetarian sushi or Fresh Mint Spring Rolls (see recipe in this chapter). It would also make an excellent marinade for a baked tofu dish.

YIELDS ⅓ CUP

¼ cup soy sauce

2 tablespoons rice vinegar

2 teaspoons sesame oil

1 teaspoon sugar

1 teaspoon minced fresh ginger

2 cloves garlic, minced and crushed

¼ teaspoon crushed red pepper flakes, or to taste

Folic Acid: only present in very small amounts

Vitamin B$_{12}$: NA

Protein:

Iron: only present in very small amounts

Zinc: only present in very small amounts

Calcium: only present in very small amounts

Vitamin D: NA

● Whisk together all ingredients.

Per Tablespoon
Calories: 29 | Fat: 2g | Sodium: 719mg | Fiber: 0g | Protein: 1g

Vegan "Pigs" in a Blanket

Use store-bought vegetarian hot dogs to make this great little appetizer that kids and adults both love. Serve with ketchup or hot mustard.

MAKES 16 "PIGS"

1 batch Quick and Easy Vegan Biscuit dough (see Chapter 3)

8 vegan hot dogs, sliced in half

Folic Acid: NA

Vitamin B$_{12}$: NA

Protein: 🌿

Iron: 🌿

Zinc: NA

Calcium: 🌿

Vitamin D: NA

1. Preheat oven to 400°F and lightly grease a baking sheet.
2. Divide dough into 16 pieces and roll into ovals.
3. Place each hot dog piece on the edge of each dough circle and wrap. Place on baking sheet. Bake for 10–12 minutes or until lightly golden brown.

Per "Pig"

Calories: 119 | Fat: 4g | Sodium: 358mg | Fiber: 1g | Protein: 7g

Party Pigs

Head to enough vegan parties, and you'll inevitably run into a variation of this recipe sooner or later—it's an old vegan favorite. If you're short on time, roll out some store-bought vegan crescent roll dough, and to try something a bit different, add a thin slice of vegan cheese or a generous sprinkle of red pepper flakes before wrapping.

Fried Zucchini Sticks

You don't have to deep-fry these zucchini sticks, just sauté them in a bit of oil if you prefer. This is a great appetizer or snack if you're craving something salty!

SERVES 4

¾ cup flour

½ teaspoon garlic powder

¾ teaspoon Italian seasoning

¼ teaspoon salt

4 zucchini, cut into strips

Oil for frying

Vegan ranch dressing or ketchup for dipping

Folic Acid: 🍎🍎

Vitamin B$_{12}$: NA

Protein: 🍎

Iron: 🍎

Zinc: 🍎

Calcium: 🍎

Vitamin D: NA

1. In a large bowl or pan, combine the flour, garlic powder, Italian seasoning, and salt.
2. Lightly toss the zucchini strips with the flour mixture, coating well.
3. Heat oil in a large skillet or frying pan. When oil is hot, gently add zucchini strips to pan.
4. Fry until lightly golden brown on all sides. Serve with vegan ranch dressing or ketchup.

Per Serving
Calories: 178 | Fat: 7g | Sodium: 166mg | Fiber: 3g | Protein: 5g

Simple Scallion Pancakes

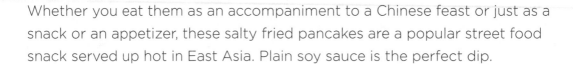

Whether you eat them as an accompaniment to a Chinese feast or just as a snack or an appetizer, these salty fried pancakes are a popular street food snack served up hot in East Asia. Plain soy sauce is the perfect dip.

YIELDS 6 LARGE PANCAKES

2 cups flour

½ teaspoon salt

2 teaspoons sesame oil, additional for brushing

¾ cup hot water

6 scallions, chopped (green parts only)

Oil for frying

Soy sauce for dipping

Folic Acid: 🍎🍎

Vitamin B₁₂: NA

Protein: 🍎

Iron: 🍎

Zinc: 🍎

Calcium: 🍎

Vitamin D: NA

① In a large bowl, combine flour and salt. Slowly add sesame oil and water, mixing, just until a dough forms. You may need a little bit less than ¾ cup water.

② Knead dough for a few minutes, then let sit for 30 minutes.

③ Divide dough into six 2" balls. Roll out each ball on a lightly floured surface. Brush with sesame oil and cover with scallions. Roll up dough and twist to form a ball. Roll out again ¼" thick.

④ Fry each pancake in hot oil 1–2 minutes on each side. Slice into squares or wedges and serve with soy sauce.

Per Pancake
Calories: 232 | Fat: 9g | Sodium: 198mg | Fiber: 2g | Protein: 5g

Walnut Asparagus "Egg" Rolls

It's not traditional, but it's certainly delicious. Spring roll wrappers or wonton wrappers are just fine if you can't find eggless egg roll wraps.

YIELDS 15 EGG ROLLS

1 bunch asparagus

2 avocados, pitted

½ onion, minced

1 teaspoon lime juice

1 tablespoon soy sauce

1 teaspoon chipotle powder

½ cup walnuts, finely chopped

¼ cup chopped fresh cilantro

15 vegan egg roll wrappers

Oil for frying

Folic Acid: 🍎

Vitamin B$_{12}$: NA

Protein: 🍎

Iron: 🍎

Zinc: 🍎

Calcium: only present in very small amounts

Vitamin D: NA

① Steam the asparagus until crisp-tender, then chop into ½" slices.

② Mash together the asparagus with the avocados, onion, lime juice, soy sauce, chipotle, walnuts, and cilantro.

③ Place 2–3 tablespoons of filling in each wrapper. Fold the bottom up, then fold the sides in, and roll, wetting the edges with water to help it stick together.

④ Fry in hot oil for 1–2 minutes on each side.

Per Egg Roll
Calories: 219 | Fat: 10g | Sodium: 209mg | Fiber: 3g | Protein: 5g

Parsley and Onion Dip

If you like packaged onion dip mixes, try this tofu-based version with fresh parsley and chives. Perfect for carrots or crackers.

SERVES 6

1 onion, chopped

3 cloves garlic, minced

1 tablespoon olive oil

1 (16-ounce) block firm tofu, well pressed

½ teaspoon onion powder

3 teaspoons lemon juice

¼ cup chopped fresh parsley

2 tablespoons chopped fresh chives

¼ teaspoon salt

Folic Acid: 🍎

Vitamin B₁₂: NA

Protein: 🍎

Iron: 🍎

Zinc: 🍎

Calcium: 🍎🍎

Vitamin D: NA

1. Sauté onions and garlic in oil for 3–4 minutes until onions are soft. Remove from heat and allow to cool slightly.
2. Process the onion and garlic with the tofu, onion powder, and lemon juice in a food processor or blender until onion is minced and tofu is almost smooth.
3. Mash together with remaining ingredients by hand.

Per Serving
Calories: 68 | Fat: 5g | Sodium: 104mg | Fiber: 1g | Protein: 5g

Tomato and Dill-Stuffed Grape Leaves (Dolmas)

Little Middle Eastern dolmas overflow with flavors and travel well in lunch boxes. Look for canned or jarred grape leaves in the ethnic aisle of your grocery store.

YIELDS ABOUT 2 DOZEN DOLMAS

3 scallions, chopped

1 tomato, diced small

¼ cup olive oil

1 cup uncooked rice

½ cup water

½ teaspoon salt

1 tablespoon chopped fresh dill

1 teaspoon dried parsley

1 tablespoon chopped fresh mint (optional)

About 40 grape leaves

Water for boiling

2 tablespoons lemon juice

Folic Acid: 🍎

Vitamin B$_{12}$: NA

Protein: 🍎

Iron: 🍎

Zinc: only present in very small amounts

Calcium: 🍎

Vitamin D: NA

1. Heat scallions and tomato in 2 tablespoons of olive oil for 2 minutes, then add rice, water, salt, dill, parsley, and mint. Cover and cook for 5 minutes. Remove from heat and cool.
2. Place about 2 teaspoons of the rice filling in the center of a grape leaf near the stem. Fold the bottom of the leaf over the filling, then fold in the sides, and roll. Continue with each grape leaf.
3. Line the bottom of a pan with extra or torn grape leaves to prevent burning. Add wrapped and filled leaves and add enough water just to cover the dolmas. Add remaining 2 tablespoons of olive oil and bring to a slow simmer.
4. Cook for 20 minutes. Drizzle with lemon juice just before serving.

Per 4 Stuffed Grape Leaves
Calories: 25 | Fat: 2g | Sodium: 163mg | Fiber: 0g | Protein: 0g

In a Hurry?

Mix together some leftover rice with vegan pesto for the filling. Wrap, simmer just a few minutes, and eat!

CHAPTER 5

Entrées

Three-Bean Casserole

If you like baked beans, you'll like this easy bean casserole. It's an easy entrée you can get in the oven in just a few minutes. Perfect for those days when all you want to do is nap!

SERVES 8

1 (15-ounce) can vegetarian baked beans

1 (15-ounce) can black beans, drained and rinsed

1 (15-ounce) can kidney beans, drained and rinsed

1 onion, chopped

⅓ cup ketchup

3 tablespoons apple cider vinegar

⅓ cup brown sugar

2 teaspoons mustard powder

2 teaspoons garlic powder

4 vegan hot dogs, cooked and chopped (optional)

Folic Acid: 🍎🍎

Vitamin B₁₂: NA

Protein: 🍎🍎

Iron: 🍎

Zinc: 🍎🍎

Calcium: 🍎

Vitamin D: NA

1. Preheat oven to 350°F.
2. Combine all ingredients except hot dogs in a large casserole dish.
3. Bake, uncovered, for 55 minutes. Add precooked vegan hot dogs just before serving.

Per Serving
Calories: 202 | Fat: 1g | Sodium: 553mg | Fiber: 10g | Protein: 10g

Barley Baked Beans

If you have a slow cooker, you can dump all the ingredients in and cook it on a medium setting for about six hours. Nothing easier than that!

SERVES 8

2 cups cooked barley

2 (15-ounce) cans pinto or navy beans, drained and rinsed

1 onion, diced

1 (28-ounce) can crushed or diced tomatoes

½ cup water

¼ cup brown sugar

⅓ cup barbecue sauce

2 tablespoons molasses

2 teaspoons mustard powder

1 teaspoon garlic powder

1 teaspoon salt, or to taste

Folic Acid: 🍎🍎

Vitamin B$_{12}$: NA

Protein: 🍎🍎

Iron: 🍎

Zinc: 🍎

Calcium: 🍎🍎

Vitamin D: NA

1. Preheat oven to 300°F.
2. In a large oiled casserole or baking dish, combine all ingredients. Cover, and bake for 2 hours, stirring occasionally.
3. Uncover and bake for 15 more minutes, or until thick and saucy.

Per Serving
Calories: 224 | Fat: 1g | Sodium: 849mg | Fiber: 9g | Protein: 8g

Chickpea Soft Tacos

For an easy and healthy taco filling wrapped up in flour tortillas, try using chickpeas! Short on time? Pick up taco seasoning packets to use instead of the spice blend—but watch out for added MSG.

SERVES 6

2 (15-ounce) cans chickpeas, drained and rinsed

½ cup water

1 (6-ounce) can tomato paste

1 tablespoon chili powder

1 teaspoon garlic powder

½ teaspoon onion powder

½ teaspoon cumin

¼ cup chopped fresh cilantro (optional)

6 flour tortillas

Optional taco fillings: shredded lettuce, black olives, vegan cheese, nondairy sour cream

Folic Acid: 🍎🍎🍎

Vitamin B$_{12}$: NA

Protein: 🍎🍎

Iron: 🍎🍎

Zinc: 🍎🍎

Calcium: 🍎🍎

Vitamin D: NA

1. In a large skillet, combine chickpeas, water, tomato paste, chili, garlic, onion powder, and cumin. Cover and simmer for 10 minutes, stirring occasionally. Uncover and simmer 1–2 minutes, until most of the liquid is absorbed.
2. Use a fork or potato masher to mash the chickpeas until half mashed. Stir in fresh cilantro if desired.
3. Spoon mixture into flour tortillas, add toppings, and wrap.

Per Serving
Calories: 285 | Fat: 4g | Sodium: 641mg | Fiber: 8g | Protein: 11g

Couscous and Bean Pilaf

This recipe is perfect as a quick lunch or dinner entrée that can be served hot or cold. Add a few extra veggies for a meal in a bowl.

SERVES 4

2 cups water or vegetable broth

2 cups couscous

2 tablespoons olive oil

2 tablespoons red wine vinegar

½ teaspoon crushed red pepper flakes

1 (15-ounce) can great Northern or cannellini beans, drained and rinsed

2 tablespoons minced pimiento peppers

2 tablespoons chopped fresh parsley

Salt and pepper, to taste

Folic Acid: 🍎🍎

Vitamin B₁₂: NA

Protein: 🍎🍎🍎

Iron: 🍎🍎

Zinc: 🍎🍎

Calcium: 🍎🍎

Vitamin D: NA

1. Bring the water or vegetable broth to a simmer; add couscous. Cover, turn off heat, and allow to sit for at least 15 minutes to cook couscous. Fluff with a fork.
2. Whisk together the olive oil, vinegar, and pepper flakes; toss with couscous.
3. Combine beans, peppers, and parsley with couscous; toss gently to combine. Season with salt and pepper.

Per Serving
Calories: 509 | Fat: 8g | Sodium: 32mg | Fiber: 10g | Protein: 19g

Italian White Beans and Rice

This is a quick, inexpensive, and hearty meal that will quickly become a favorite standby on busy nights. It's nutritious, filling, and can easily be doubled for a crowd.

SERVES 4

½ onion, diced

2 ribs celery, diced

3 cloves garlic, minced

2 tablespoons olive oil

1 (14-ounce) can diced or crushed tomatoes

1 (15-ounce) can cannellini or great Northern beans, drained and rinsed

½ teaspoon parsley

½ teaspoon basil

1 cup rice, cooked

1 tablespoon balsamic vinegar

Folic Acid: 🍎🍎🍎

Vitamin B$_{12}$: NA

Protein: 🍎🍎

Iron: 🍎🍎

Zinc: 🍎🍎

Calcium: 🍎🍎

Vitamin D: NA

1. Sauté onion, celery, and garlic in olive oil for 3–5 minutes, until onion and celery are soft.
2. Reduce heat to medium-low and add tomatoes, beans, parsley, and basil. Cover, and simmer for 10 minutes, stirring occasionally.
3. Stir in cooked rice and balsamic vinegar; cook, uncovered, a few more minutes, until liquid is absorbed.

Per Serving
Calories: 325 | Fat: 8g | Sodium: 135mg | Fiber: 8g | Protein: 12g

Macro-Inspired Veggie Bowl

Truly nourishing, this is a full meal in a bowl, inspired by macrobiotic cuisine.

SERVES 6

2 cups brown rice, cooked

1 batch Sesame Baked Tofu (Chapter 5), chopped into cubes

1 head broccoli, steamed and chopped

1 red or yellow bell pepper, sliced thin

1 cup Goddess Dressing (Chapter 7)

½ cup pumpkin seeds or sunflower seeds

2 teaspoons dulse or kelp seaweed flakes (optional)

Folic Acid: 🍎🍎

Vitamin B$_{12}$: NA

Protein: 🍎🍎🍎

Iron: 🍎🍎🍎

Zinc: 🍎🍎

Calcium: 🍎🍎🍎

Vitamin D: NA

1. Divide brown rice into 6 bowls.
2. Top each bowl with Sesame Baked Tofu, broccoli, and bell pepper.
3. Drizzle with dressing, and sprinkle with seeds and seaweed flakes.

Per Serving
Calories: 547 | Fat: 37g | Sodium: 911 | Fiber: 11g | Protein: 28g

Quinoa and Hummus Sandwich Wrap

Lunch is the perfect time to fill up on whole grains. If you have leftover tabbouleh, use that in place of the cooked quinoa.

SERVES 1

1 tortilla or flavored wrap, warmed

3 tablespoons hummus

⅓ cup cooked quinoa

½ teaspoon lemon juice

2 teaspoons Italian or vinaigrette salad dressing

1 roasted red pepper, sliced into strips

Folic Acid: 🍎🍎

Vitamin B$_{12}$: NA

Protein: 🍎🍎

Iron: 🍎🍎

Zinc: 🍎🍎

Calcium: 🍎

Vitamin D: NA

1. Spread warmed tortilla with a layer of hummus, then quinoa; drizzle with lemon juice and salad dressing.
2. Layer red pepper on top; wrap.

Per Serving
Calories: 332 | Fat: 12g | Sodium: 627mg | Fiber: 6g | Protein: 11g

Five-Minute Vegan Pasta Salad

Once you have the pasta cooked and cooled, this pasta salad takes just five minutes to assemble, as it's made with store-bought dressing. A balsamic vinaigrette or tomato dressing would also work well.

SERVES 4

4 cups cooked pasta

¾ cup vegan Italian salad dressing

3 scallions, chopped

½ cup sliced black olives

1 tomato, chopped

1 avocado, diced (optional)

Salt and pepper, to taste

Folic Acid: 🍎

Vitamin B$_{12}$: NA

Protein: 🍎🍎

Iron: 🍎🍎

Zinc: 🍎

Calcium: 🍎

Vitamin D: NA

● Toss together all ingredients. Chill for at least 1½ hours before serving, if time allows, to let flavors combine.

Per Serving
Calories: 378 | Fat: 16g | Sodium: 877mg | Fiber: 4g | Protein: 9g

Pasta and Peas

If you're not feeling the peas in this recipe, just use artichoke hearts or broccoli, or any frozen mixed veggies you like.

SERVES 6

1½ cups plain or unsweetened fortified soymilk

1 teaspoon garlic powder

2 tablespoons vegan margarine

1 tablespoon flour

1½ cups green peas, fresh or frozen, thawed

⅓ cup nutritional yeast

1 (12-ounce) package pasta, cooked

Salt and pepper, to taste

Folic Acid: 🍏🍏🍏

Vitamin B$_{12}$: 🍏🍏🍏

Protein: 🍏🍏

Iron: 🍏🍏

Zinc: 🍏🍏

Calcium: 🍏

Vitamin D: 🍏

1. In a medium pot, whisk together the soymilk, garlic powder, and margarine over low heat. Add flour; stir well to combine, heating just until thickened, about 5 minutes.
2. Add peas and nutritional yeast and stir until heated and well mixed, about 5 minutes; pour over pasta.
3. Season with salt and pepper, to taste.

Per Serving
Calories: 312 | Fat: 6g | Sodium: 124mg | Fiber: 4g | Protein: 13g

Easy Fried Tofu

This recipe makes a simple fried tofu that you can serve with just about any dipping sauce for a snack, or add to salads or stir-fries instead of plain tofu.

SERVES 3

1 (16-ounce) block firm or extra-firm tofu, cubed

¼ cup soy sauce (optional)

2 tablespoons flour

2 tablespoons nutritional yeast

1 teaspoon garlic powder

¼ teaspoon salt, or to taste

Dash pepper

Oil for frying

Folic Acid: 🍎🍎🍎

Vitamin B$_{12}$: 🍎🍎🍎

Protein: 🍎🍎

Iron: 🍎

Zinc: 🍎

Calcium: 🍎

Vitamin D: NA

1. Marinate sliced tofu in soy sauce in the refrigerator for at least 1 hour. This step is optional.
2. In a small bowl, combine flour, yeast, garlic powder, salt, and pepper.
3. Coat tofu well with flour mixture on all sides.
4. Fry in hot oil until crispy and lightly golden brown on all sides, about 4–5 minutes.

Per Serving
Calories: 232 | Fat: 19g | Sodium: 208mg | Fiber: 2g | Protein: 11g

Eggless Egg Salad

Vegan egg salad looks just like the real thing and is much quicker to make. Use this recipe to make egg salad sandwiches, or serve it on a bed of lettuce with tomato slices and enjoy it just as it is.

SERVES 4

1 (16-ounce) block firm tofu, lightly steamed and cooled

1 (12-ounce) block silken tofu

½ cup vegan mayonnaise

⅓ cup sweet pickle relish

¾ teaspoon apple cider vinegar

½ rib celery, diced

2 tablespoons minced onion

1½ tablespoons Dijon mustard

2 tablespoons chopped chives (optional)

2 tablespoons vegan bacon bits (optional)

1 teaspoon paprika

Folic Acid: 🍎

Vitamin B$_{12}$: NA

Protein: 🍎🍎

Iron: 🍎

Zinc: 🍎🍎

Calcium: 🍎🍎

Vitamin D: NA

1. In a medium-size bowl, use a fork to mash the tofu together with the rest of the ingredients, except the bacon bits and paprika.
2. Chill for at least 15 minutes before serving to allow flavors to mingle.
3. Garnish with bacon bits and paprika just before serving.

Per Serving
Calories: 318 | Fat: 24g | Sodium: 428mg | Fiber: 2g | Protein: 11g

Black and Green-Veggie Burritos

These black bean burritos, filled with zucchini or yellow summer squash, are quick and easy. Just add in the fixings—salsa, avocado slices, some nondairy sour cream—the works!

SERVES 4

1 onion, chopped

2 zucchini or yellow squash, cut into thin strips

1 bell pepper, any color, chopped

2 tablespoons olive oil

½ teaspoon oregano

½ teaspoon cumin

1 (15-ounce) can black beans, drained and rinsed

1 (4-ounce) can green chilies

1 cup cooked rice

4 large flour tortillas, warmed

Folic Acid: 🍎🍎🍎

Vitamin B$_{12}$: NA

Protein: 🍎🍎🍎

Iron: 🍎🍎

Zinc: 🍎🍎

Calcium: 🍎🍎

Vitamin D: NA

1. Heat onion, zucchini, and bell pepper in olive oil until vegetables are soft, about 4–5 minutes.
2. Reduce heat to low and add oregano, cumin, black beans, and chilies; combine well. Cook, stirring, until well combined and heated through.
3. Place ¼ cup rice in the center of each flour tortilla and top with the bean mixture. Fold the bottom of the tortilla up, then snugly wrap one side, then the other.
4. Serve as is, or bake in a 350°F oven for 15 minutes for a crispy burrito.

Per Serving
Calories: 377 | Fat: 10g | Sodium: 554mg | Fiber: 13g | Protein: 15g

Barley Pilaf with Edamame and Roasted Red Peppers

Don't forget: Freshly ground pepper will give the best flavor to all your recipes, including this one. Serve chilled like a salad, or heat the edamame lightly first for a warmed and high-protein pilaf.

SERVES 6

2 cups frozen shelled edamame, thawed and drained

2 cups cooked barley

½ cup chopped roasted red peppers

⅔ cup green peas, fresh or frozen, thawed

⅔ cup corn, fresh, canned, or frozen, thawed

1½ tablespoons Dijon mustard

2 tablespoons lemon or lime juice

¾ teaspoon garlic powder

2 tablespoons olive oil

Salt and pepper, to taste

¼ cup chopped fresh cilantro

1 avocado, diced (optional)

Folic Acid: 🍎
Vitamin B$_{12}$: NA
Protein: 🍎🍎
Iron: 🍎
Zinc: 🍎
Calcium: 🍎
Vitamin D: NA

1. In a large bowl, combine the edamame, barley, peppers, peas, and corn.
2. In a separate small bowl, whisk together the mustard, lemon or lime juice, garlic powder, and olive oil. Drizzle over barley mixture; toss gently to coat well.
3. Season with salt and pepper and toss lightly with cilantro and avocado.

Per Serving
Calories: 190 | Fat: 4g | Sodium: 100mg | Fiber: 9g | Protein: 9g

Curried Rice and Lentils

With no added fat, this is a very simple one-pot side dish or starter recipe. Personalize it with some chopped greens, browned seitan, or a veggie mix.

SERVES 4

1½ cups white rice, uncooked

1 cup lentils, uncooked

2 tomatoes, diced

3½ cups water or vegetable broth

1 bay leaf (optional)

1 tablespoon curry powder

½ teaspoon cumin

½ teaspoon turmeric

½ teaspoon garlic powder

Salt and pepper, to taste

Folic Acid: 🍎🍎🍎

Vitamin B$_{12}$: NA

Protein: 🍎🍎🍎

Iron: 🍎🍎🍎

Zinc: 🍎🍎🍎

Calcium: 🍎

Vitamin D: NA

1. In a large soup or stockpot, combine all ingredients except salt and pepper. Bring to a slow simmer, then cover and cook for 20 minutes, stirring occasionally, until rice is done and liquid is absorbed.
2. Taste, then add salt and pepper as desired. Remove bay leaf before serving.

Per Serving
Calories: 436 | Fat: 1g | Sodium: 13mg | Fiber: 17g | Protein: 18g

Peanut Butter Noodles

Drown your noodles in this mildly flavored peanut butter sauce recipe. Who doesn't love peanut butter?

SERVES 4

1 pound Asian-style noodles or regular pasta

⅓ cup peanut butter

⅓ cup water

3 tablespoons soy sauce

2 tablespoons lime juice

2 tablespoons rice vinegar

1 tablespoon sesame oil

½ teaspoon ginger powder

1 teaspoon sugar

½ teaspoon crushed red pepper flakes (optional)

Folic Acid: 🍎🍎🍎

Vitamin B$_{12}$: NA

Protein: 🍎🍎🍎

Iron: 🍎🍎

Zinc: 🍎🍎🍎

Calcium: 🍎

Vitamin D: NA

1. Prepare noodles or pasta according to package instructions and set aside.
2. Whisk together remaining ingredients over low heat just until combined, about 3 minutes. Toss with noodles.

Per Serving
Calories: 584 | Fat: 16g | Sodium: 782mg | Fiber: 5g | Protein: 21g

Balsamic Dijon Orzo

Defying logic, this simple dish flavored with balsamic and Dijon is somehow exponentially greater than the sum of its parts. Add a dash of sugar or agave if you find the tangy Dijon overpowering.

SERVES 4

3 tablespoons balsamic vinegar

1½ tablespoons Dijon mustard

1½ tablespoons olive oil

1 teaspoon basil

1 teaspoon parsley

½ teaspoon oregano

1½ cups orzo, cooked

2 medium tomatoes, chopped

½ cup sliced black olives

1 (15-ounce) can great Northern or cannellini beans, drained and rinsed

½ teaspoon salt, or to taste

¼ teaspoon pepper

Folic Acid: 🍎🍎🍎

Vitamin B$_{12}$: NA

Protein: 🍎🍎

Iron: 🍎🍎🍎

Zinc: 🍎🍎

Calcium: 🍎🍎

Vitamin D: NA

1. In a small bowl or container, whisk together the vinegar, mustard, olive oil, basil, parsley, and oregano until well mixed.
2. Over low heat, combine the orzo with the balsamic dressing; add tomatoes, olives, and beans. Cook for 3–4 minutes, stirring to combine.
3. Season with salt and pepper.

Per Serving
Calories: 356 | Fat: 8g | Sodium: 505mg | Fiber: 8g | Protein: 14g

Creamy Sun-Dried Tomato Pasta

Silken tofu makes a creamy low-fat sauce base. If using dried tomatoes rather than oil-packed, be sure to rehydrate them well first.

SERVES 6

1 (12-ounce) block silken tofu, drained

¼ cup soymilk

2 tablespoons red wine vinegar

½ teaspoon garlic powder

½ teaspoon salt, or to taste

1¼ cups sun-dried tomatoes, rehydrated

1 teaspoon parsley

1 (12-ounce) package pasta, cooked

2 tablespoons chopped fresh basil

Folic Acid: 🍎🍎🍎

Vitamin B₁₂: 🍎

Protein: 🍎🍎

Iron: 🍎🍎

Zinc: 🍎🍎

Calcium: 🍎

Vitamin D: only present in very small amounts

1. In a blender or food processor, blend together the tofu, soymilk, vinegar, garlic powder, and salt until smooth and creamy. Add tomatoes and parsley; pulse until tomatoes are finely diced.
2. Transfer sauce to a small pot and heat over medium-low heat just until hot, about 5–10 minutes.
3. Pour sauce over pasta and sprinkle with fresh chopped basil.

Per Serving
Calories: 274 | Fat: 3g | Sodium: 441mg | Fiber: 3g | Protein: 12g

Lemon Basil Tofu

Moist and chewy, this zesty baked tofu is reminiscent of lemon chicken. Serve over steamed rice with extra marinade.

SERVES 6

3 tablespoons lemon juice

1 tablespoon soy sauce

2 teaspoons apple cider vinegar

1 tablespoon Dijon mustard

¾ teaspoon sugar

3 tablespoons olive oil

2 tablespoons chopped basil, plus extra for garnish

2 (16-ounce) blocks firm or extra-firm tofu, well pressed

Folic Acid: only present in very small amounts

Vitamin B₁₂: NA

Protein: 🍎🍎

Iron: 🍎

Zinc: 🍎

Calcium: 🍎

Vitamin D: NA

1. Whisk together all ingredients except tofu; transfer to a baking dish or casserole pan.
2. Slice the tofu into ½"-thick strips or triangles.
3. Place the tofu in the marinade and coat well. Allow to marinate in the refrigerator for at least 1 hour or overnight, making sure tofu is well coated in marinade.
4. Preheat oven to 350°F.
5. Bake for 15 minutes, turn over, then bake for another 10–12 minutes, or until done. Garnish with a few extra bits of chopped fresh basil.

Per Serving
Calories: 148 | Fat: 10g | Sodium: 226mg | Fiber: 0g | Protein: 9g

Mexico City Protein Bowl

A quick meal in a bowl, this dish is reminiscent of Mexico City street food stalls, but healthier for you and your baby-to-be!

SERVES 2

½ (16-ounce) block firm tofu, diced small

1 scallion, chopped

1 tablespoon olive oil

½ cup peas, fresh or frozen, thawed

½ cup corn kernels, fresh, canned, or frozen, thawed

½ teaspoon chili powder

1 (15-ounce) can black beans, drained and rinsed

2 corn tortillas

Hot sauce, to taste

Folic Acid: 🍎🍎🍎

Vitamin B₁₂: NA

Protein: 🍎🍎🍎

Iron: 🍎🍎🍎

Zinc: 🍎🍎🍎

Calcium: 🍎🍎

Vitamin D: NA

1. Heat tofu and scallion in olive oil for 2–3 minutes; add peas, corn, and chili powder. Cook another 1–2 minutes, stirring frequently.
2. Reduce heat to medium-low; add black beans. Heat for 4–5 minutes, until well combined and heated through.
3. Place a corn tortilla in the bottom of a bowl; spoon ½ the beans and tofu over the top of each. Season with hot sauce, to taste.

Per Serving
Calories: 518 | Fat: 12g | Sodium: 593mg | Fiber: 23g | Protein: 31g

Pineapple-Glazed Tofu

If you like sweet and sour dishes, try this saucy, sweet, Pineapple-Glazed Tofu. Toss with some noodles, or add some diced veggies to make it an entrée.

SERVES 3

½ cup pineapple preserves

2 tablespoons balsamic vinegar

2 tablespoons soy sauce

⅔ cup pineapple juice

1 (16-ounce) block firm or extra-firm tofu, cubed

3 tablespoons flour

2 tablespoons oil

1 teaspoon cornstarch

Folic Acid: 🍎

Vitamin B₁₂: NA

Protein: 🍎🍎

Iron: 🍎

Zinc: 🍎

Calcium: 🍎

Vitamin D: NA

1. Whisk together the preserves, vinegar, soy sauce, and pineapple juice.
2. Coat tofu in flour, then sauté in oil for 1–2 minutes, until lightly golden.
3. Reduce heat to medium-low; add pineapple sauce, stirring well to combine and coat tofu.
4. Heat for 3–4 minutes, stirring frequently, then add cornstarch, whisking to combine and avoid lumps. Heat for a few more minutes, stirring, until sauce has thickened.

Per Serving
Calories: 366 | Fat: 13g | Sodium: 673mg | Fiber: 1g | Protein: 11g

Tandoori Seitan

You can enjoy the flavors of traditional Indian tandoori without firing up your grill by simmering the seitan on the stove top.

SERVES 6

⅔ cup plain soy yogurt

2 tablespoons lemon juice

1½ tablespoons tandoori spice blend

½ teaspoon cumin

½ teaspoon garlic powder

¼ teaspoon salt, or to taste

1 (16-ounce) package prepared seitan, chopped

1 bell pepper, chopped

1 onion, chopped

1 tomato, chopped

2 tablespoons oil

Folic Acid: only present in very small amounts

Vitamin B$_{12}$: NA

Protein: 🌶🌶🌶

Iron: 🌶

Zinc: only present in very small amounts

Calcium: 🌶

Vitamin D: 🌶

1. In a shallow bowl or pan, whisk together the yogurt, lemon juice, and all the spices; add seitan. Allow to marinate in the refrigerator for at least 1 hour. Reserve marinade.
2. Sauté pepper, onion, and tomato in oil until just barely soft.
3. Reduce heat to low; add seitan. Cook, tossing seitan occasionally, for 8–10 minutes.
4. Serve topped with extra marinade.

Per Serving
Calories: 148 | Fat: 6g | Sodium: 419mg | Fiber: 2g | Protein: 16g

Stove Top Cheater's Mac 'n' Cheese

Yes, it's cheating just a little to make vegan macaroni and cheese starting with store-bought "cheese," but who cares? The secret to getting this recipe super creamy and cheesy is using cream cheese as well as vegan Cheddar. It's not particularly healthy, but at least it's still cholesterol free!

SERVES 6

1 (12-ounce) package macaroni

1 cup plain or unsweetened fortified soymilk

2 tablespoons vegan margarine

½ teaspoon onion powder

1 teaspoon garlic powder

½ cup vegan cream cheese

½ cup vegan Cheddar cheese, grated

⅓ cup nutritional yeast

½ teaspoon salt, or to taste

Black pepper, to taste

Folic Acid: 🍎🍎🍎

Vitamin B$_{12}$: 🍎🍎🍎

Protein: 🍎🍎

Iron: 🍎

Zinc: 🍎🍎

Calcium: 🍎🍎

Vitamin D: 🍎

1. Prepare macaroni according to package instructions. Drain well and return to pot.
2. Over low heat, stir in soymilk and vegan margarine until melted.
3. Add remaining ingredients, stirring to combine over low heat, until cheese is melted and ingredients are well mixed, about 5–10 minutes.

Per Serving
Calories: 411 | Fat: 13g | Sodium: 549mg | Fiber: 3g | Protein: 13g

Sweet and Spicy Peanut Noodles

Like the call of the siren, these noodles entice you with their sweet pineapple flavor, then scorch your tongue with fiery chilies. Very sneaky, indeed.

SERVES 4

1 (12-ounce) package Asian-style noodles

⅓ cup peanut butter

2 tablespoons soy sauce

⅔ cup pineapple juice

2 cloves garlic, minced

1 teaspoon grated fresh ginger

½ teaspoon salt, or to taste

1 tablespoon olive oil

1 teaspoon sesame oil

2–3 small chilies, minced

¾ cup diced pineapple, fresh or canned

Folic Acid: 🍎

Vitamin B₁₂: NA

Protein: 🍎 🍎

Iron: 🍎

Zinc: 🍎

Calcium: 🍎

Vitamin D: NA

1. Prepare noodles according to package instructions and set aside.
2. In a small saucepan over low heat, stir together the peanut butter, soy sauce, pineapple juice, garlic, ginger, and salt just until well combined, about 5 minutes.
3. In a large skillet, heat the oils; fry chilies and pineapple, stirring frequently, until pineapple is lightly browned, about 2–3 minutes. Add noodles; fry for another minute, stirring well.
4. Reduce heat to low and add peanut butter sauce mixture; stir to combine well. Heat for 1 more minute.

Per Serving
Calories: 329 | Fat: 16g | Sodium: 977mg | Fiber: 2g | Protein: 10g

Pineapple TVP Baked Beans

Add a kick to these saucy homemade vegetarian baked beans with a bit of cayenne pepper if you'd like.

SERVES 4

2 (15-ounce) cans pinto or navy beans, partially drained

1 onion, diced

⅔ cup vegan barbecue sauce

2 tablespoons prepared mustard

2 tablespoons brown sugar

1 cup TVP

1 cup hot water

1 (8-ounce) can diced pineapple, drained

¾ teaspoon salt, or to taste

½ teaspoon pepper

Folic Acid: 🍎🍎🍎

Vitamin B₁₂: NA

Protein: 🍎🍎🍎

Iron: 🍎🍎

Zinc: 🍎🍎

Calcium: 🍎🍎

Vitamin D: NA

1. In a large stockpot, combine beans and about half their liquid, onion, barbecue sauce, mustard, and brown sugar; bring to a slow simmer. Cover and allow to cook for at least 10 minutes, stirring occasionally.
2. Combine TVP with hot water; allow to sit for 6–8 minutes to rehydrate TVP. Drain.
3. Add TVP, pineapple, salt, and pepper to beans; cover and slowly simmer another 10–12 minutes.

Per Serving
Calories: 389 | Fat: 2g | Sodium: 1,461mg | Fiber: 15g | Protein: 23g

Tofu "Chicken" Nuggets

Try dipping these nuggets into ketchup or a sweet and sour sauce.

SERVES 4

¼ cup plain or unsweetened fortified soymilk

2 tablespoons prepared mustard

3 tablespoons nutritional yeast

½ cup bread crumbs

½ cup flour

1 teaspoon poultry seasoning

1 teaspoon garlic powder

1 teaspoon onion powder

½ teaspoon salt, or to taste

¼ teaspoon pepper

1 (16-ounce) block firm or extra-firm tofu, sliced into thin strips

Oil for frying (optional)

Folic Acid: 🍎🍎
Vitamin B$_{12}$: 🍎🍎🍎
Protein: 🍎🍎
Iron: 🍎
Zinc: 🍎🍎
Calcium: 🍎
Vitamin D: only present in very small amounts

1. In a large shallow pan, whisk together the soymilk, mustard, and nutritional yeast.
2. In a separate bowl, combine the bread crumbs, flour, poultry seasoning, garlic, onion powder, salt, and pepper.
3. Coat each piece of tofu with the soymilk mixture, then coat well in bread crumbs and flour mixture.
4. Fry in hot oil until lightly golden brown, about 3–4 minutes on each side, or bake in 375°F oven for 20 minutes, turning once.

Per Serving
Calories: 135 | Fat: 4g | Sodium: 518mg | Fiber: 1g | Protein: 10g

The Easiest Black Bean Burger Recipe in the World

Veggie burgers are notorious for falling apart. If you're sick of crumbly burgers, try this simple method for making black bean patties. It's 100 percent guaranteed to stick together.

YIELDS 6 PATTIES

1 (15-ounce) can black beans, drained and rinsed

3 tablespoons minced onion

1 teaspoon salt, or to taste

1½ teaspoons garlic powder

2 teaspoons parsley

1 teaspoon chili powder

⅔ cup flour

Oil for pan frying

Folic Acid: 🍎🍎🍎

Vitamin B$_{12}$: NA

Protein: 🍎🍎

Iron: 🍎

Zinc: 🍎

Calcium: 🍎

Vitamin D: NA

1. In a blender or food processor, process the black beans until halfway mashed, or mash with a fork.
2. Remove to a bowl and add onions, salt, garlic powder, parsley, and chili powder and mash to combine.
3. Add flour, a bit at time, again mashing together to combine. You may need a little bit more or less than ⅔ cup. Beans should stick together completely.
4. Form into patties and pan fry in a bit of oil for 2–3 minutes on each side. Patties will appear to be done on the outside while still a bit mushy on the inside, so fry them a few minutes longer than you think they need.

Per Patty
Calories: 210 | Fat: 8g | Sodium: 559mg | Fiber: 7g | Protein: 8g

Easy Falafel Patties

Natural food stores sell a vegan instant falafel mix, but it doesn't take very much work at all to make your own from scratch.

SERVES 4

1 (15-ounce) can chickpeas, well drained and rinsed

½ onion, minced

1 tablespoon flour

1 teaspoon cumin

¾ teaspoon garlic powder

¾ teaspoon salt, or to taste

Egg substitute for 1 egg

¼ cup chopped fresh parsley

2 tablespoons chopped fresh cilantro (optional)

Folic Acid: 🍎🍎

Vitamin B$_{12}$: NA

Protein: 🍎

Iron: 🍎

Zinc: 🍎🍎

Calcium: 🍎

Vitamin D: NA

1. Preheat oven to 375°F.
2. Place chickpeas in a large bowl and mash with a fork until coarsely mashed, or pulse in a food processor until chopped.
3. Combine chickpeas with onion, flour, cumin, garlic powder, salt, and egg substitute; mash together to combine. Add parsley and cilantro.
4. Shape mixture into 2" balls or 1"-thick patties and bake on lightly oiled baking sheet in oven for 15 minutes, or until crisp. Falafel can also be fried in oil for about 5–6 minutes on each side.

Per Serving
Calories: 141 | Fat: 1g | Sodium: 752mg | Fiber: 5g | Protein: 6g

Tofu BBQ Sauce "Steaks"

These chewy tofu "steaks" have a hearty texture and a meaty flavor. It's delicious as is, or add it to a sandwich. If you're in a rush, this is a super-easy foolproof recipe.

SERVES 6

⅓ cup vegan barbecue sauce

¼ cup water

2 teaspoons balsamic vinegar

2 tablespoons soy sauce

1–2 tablespoons hot sauce, or to taste

2 teaspoons sugar

2 (16-ounce) blocks firm or extra-firm tofu, well pressed

½ onion, chopped

2 tablespoons olive oil

Folic Acid: only present in very small amounts

Vitamin B$_{12}$: NA

Protein: 🍎 🍎

Iron: 🍎

Zinc: 🍎

Calcium: 🍎

Vitamin D: NA

1. In a small bowl, whisk together the barbecue sauce, water, vinegar, soy sauce, hot sauce, and sugar until well combined. Set aside.
2. Slice tofu into ¼"-thick strips.
3. Sauté onion in oil; carefully add tofu. Fry tofu on both sides until lightly golden brown, about 2 minutes on each side.
4. Reduce heat; add barbecue sauce mixture, stirring to coat tofu well. Cook over medium-low heat until sauce absorbs and thickens, about 5–6 minutes.

Per Serving
Calories: 155 | Fat: 8g | Sodium: 522mg | Fiber: 0g | Protein: 9g

Lentil and Rice Loaf

Made from two of the cheapest ingredients on the planet, this recipe is great if you're saving up for that fancy baby bedroom set. Serve with mashed potatoes and gravy for an all-American meal. Use poultry seasoning in place of the individual herbs, if you prefer.

SERVES 6

3 cloves garlic

1 large onion, diced

2 tablespoons oil

3½ cups cooked lentils

2¼ cups cooked rice

⅓ cup plus 3 tablespoons ketchup

2 tablespoons flour

Egg replacer for 1 egg

½ teaspoon parsley

½ teaspoon thyme

½ teaspoon oregano

¼ teaspoon sage

¾ teaspoon salt, or to taste

½ teaspoon black pepper

Folic Acid: 🍎🍎🍎
Vitamin B$_{12}$: NA
Protein: 🍎🍎
Iron: 🍎🍎
Zinc: 🍎🍎
Calcium: 🍎
Vitamin D: NA

1. Preheat oven to 350°F.
2. Sauté garlic and onions in oil until onions are soft and translucent, about 3–4 minutes.
3. In a large bowl, use a fork or a potato masher to mash the lentils until about ⅔ mashed.
4. Add garlic and onions, rice, ⅓ cup ketchup, and flour; combine well. Add egg replacer and remaining seasoning; mash to combine.
5. Gently press the mixture into a lightly greased loaf pan. Drizzle the remaining 3 tablespoons ketchup on top.
6. Bake for 60 minutes. Allow to cool at least 10 minutes before serving, as loaf will firm slightly as it cools.

Per Serving
Calories: 295 | Fat: 5g | Sodium: 528mg | Fiber: 10g | Protein: 13g

Basic Tofu Lasagna

Seasoned tofu takes the place of ricotta cheese in this recipe, and really does look and taste like the real thing. Fresh parsley adds flavor, and with store-bought sauce, it's quick to get in the oven.

SERVES 6

1 (16-ounce) block firm tofu

1 (12-ounce) block silken tofu

¼ cup nutritional yeast

1 tablespoon lemon juice

1 tablespoon soy sauce

1 teaspoon garlic powder

2 teaspoons basil

3 tablespoons chopped fresh parsley

1 teaspoon salt, or to taste

4 cups vegan spaghetti sauce

1 (16-ounce) package lasagna noodles, cooked

Folic Acid: 🍎 🍎 🍎

Vitamin B$_{12}$: 🍎 🍎 🍎

Protein: 🍎 🍎 🍎

Iron: 🍎 🍎

Zinc: 🍎 🍎 🍎

Calcium: 🍎 🍎

Vitamin D: NA

1. Preheat oven to 350°F.
2. In a large bowl, mash together the firm tofu, silken tofu, nutritional yeast, lemon juice, soy sauce, garlic powder, basil, parsley, and salt until combined and crumbly like ricotta cheese.
3. To assemble the lasagna, spread about ⅔ cup spaghetti sauce on the bottom of a lasagna pan, then add a layer of noodles.
4. Spread about ½ the tofu mixture on top of the noodles, followed by another layer of sauce. Place a second layer of noodles on top, followed by the remaining tofu and more sauce. Finish it off with a third layer of noodles and the rest of the sauce.
5. Cover and bake for 25 minutes.

Per Serving
Calories: 520 | Fat: 9g | Sodium: 1,273mg | Fiber: 8g | Protein: 22g

Easy Pad Thai Noodles

Volumes could be written about Thailand's national dish. It's sweet, sour, spicy, and salty all at once, and filled with as much texture and flavor as the streets of Bangkok themselves.

SERVES 4

1 pound thin rice noodles

¼ cup tahini

¼ cup ketchup

¼ cup soy sauce

2 tablespoons white, rice, or cider vinegar

3 tablespoons lime juice

2 tablespoons sugar

¾ teaspoon crushed red pepper flakes or cayenne

1 (16-ounce) block firm or extra-firm tofu, diced small

3 cloves garlic, minced

¼ cup vegetable or safflower oil

4 scallions, chopped

½ teaspoon salt, or to taste

Optional toppings: extra scallions, crushed toasted peanuts, sliced lime

Folic Acid: 🍎

Vitamin B₁₂: NA

Protein: 🍎🍎

Iron: 🍎🍎

Zinc: 🍎🍎

Calcium: 🍎🍎

Vitamin D: NA

1. Cover the noodles in hot water and set aside to soak until soft, about 5 minutes.
2. Whisk together the tahini, ketchup, soy sauce, vinegar, lime juice, sugar, and pepper flakes.
3. In a large skillet, fry the tofu and garlic in oil until tofu is lightly golden brown, about 8–10 minutes. Add drained noodles, stirring to combine well; fry for 2–3 minutes. Reduce heat to medium; add tahini and ketchup mixture, stirring well to combine. Allow to cook for 3–4 minutes, until well combined and heated through. Add scallions and salt and heat 1 more minute, stirring well.
4. Serve with extra chopped scallions, crushed peanuts, and a lime wedge or two.

Per Serving
Calories: 718 | Fat: 25g | Sodium: 1,401mg | Fiber: 3g | Protein: 11g

Spaghetti with Italian "Meatballs"

These little TVP nuggets are so chewy and addictive, you just might want to make a double batch. If you can't find beef-flavored bouillon, just use what you have on hand. Don't be tempted to add extra water to the TVP, as it needs to be a little dry for this recipe.

SERVES 6

½ vegetarian beef-flavored bouillon cube (optional)

⅔ cup hot water

⅔ cup TVP

Egg replacer for 2 eggs

½ onion, minced

2 tablespoons ketchup or vegan barbecue sauce

½ teaspoon garlic powder

1 teaspoon basil

1 teaspoon parsley

½ teaspoon sage

½ teaspoon salt, or to taste

½ cup bread crumbs

⅔–¾ cup flour

Oil for pan frying

3 cups prepared vegan spaghetti sauce

1 (12-ounce) package spaghetti noodles, cooked

Folic Acid: 🍎🍎🍎

Vitamin B₁₂: NA

Protein: 🍎🍎🍎

Iron: 🍎🍎

Zinc: 🍎🍎

Calcium: 🍎🍎

Vitamin D: NA

1. Dissolve bouillon cube in hot water; pour over TVP to reconstitute. Allow to sit for 6–7 minutes. Gently press to remove any excess moisture.
2. In a large bowl, combine the TVP, egg replacer, onion, ketchup, and seasonings until well mixed.
3. Add bread crumbs; combine well. Add flour, a few tablespoons at a time, mixing well to combine, until mixture is sticky and thick. You may need a little more or less than ⅔ cup.
4. Using lightly floured hands, shape into balls 1½"–2" thick.
5. Pan fry "meatballs" in a bit of oil over medium heat, rolling them around in the pan to maintain the shape, until golden brown on all sides, about 10 minutes.
6. Reduce heat to medium-low; add spaghetti sauce and heat thoroughly. Serve over noodles.

Per Serving
Calories: 495 | Fat: 9g | Sodium: 850mg | Fiber: 8g | Protein: 18g

Braised Tofu and Veggie Cacciatore

This cacciatore is incredibly versatile! Serve over pasta or try it with rice, whole grains, or even baked potatoes or polenta.

SERVES 4

½ yellow onion, chopped

½ cup sliced mushrooms

1 carrot, chopped

3 cloves garlic, minced

2 (16-ounce) blocks firm or extra-firm tofu, chopped into cubes

2 tablespoons olive oil

1½ cups vegetable broth

1 (14-ounce) can diced tomatoes or 3 large fresh tomatoes, diced

1 (6-ounce) can tomato paste

1 bay leaf (optional)

½ teaspoon salt, or to taste

1 teaspoon parsley

1 teaspoon basil

1 teaspoon oregano

Folic Acid: 🍎
Vitamin B$_{12}$: NA
Protein: 🍎🍎🍎
Iron: 🍎🍎
Zinc: 🍎🍎
Calcium: 🍎🍎
Vitamin D: only present in very small amounts

1. Sauté the onion, mushrooms, carrot, garlic, and tofu in olive oil for 4–5 minutes, stirring frequently.
2. Reduce heat to medium-low; add vegetable broth, tomatoes, tomato paste, bay leaf, salt, and spices.
3. Cover, and allow to simmer for 20 minutes, stirring occasionally. Remove bay leaf before serving.

Per Serving
Calories: 256 | Fat: 14g | Sodium: 845mg | Fiber: 6g | Protein: 17g

Orange-Glazed "Chicken" Tofu

If you're craving Chinese restaurant–style orange-glazed chicken, try this easy tofu version. It's slightly sweet, slightly salty, and, if you add some crushed red pepper, it'll have a bit of spice as well! Double the sauce and add some veggies for a full meal over rice.

SERVES 3

⅔ cup orange juice

2 tablespoons soy sauce

2 tablespoons rice vinegar

1 tablespoon maple syrup

½ teaspoon red pepper flakes (optional)

2 tablespoons olive oil

1 (16-ounce) block firm or extra-firm tofu, well pressed and chopped into 1" cubes

3 cloves garlic, minced

1½ teaspoons cornstarch

2 tablespoons water

Folic Acid: 🍎

Vitamin B$_{12}$: NA

Protein: 🍎🍎

Iron: 🍎

Zinc: 🍎🍎

Calcium: 🍎

Vitamin D: NA

① Whisk together the orange juice, soy sauce, vinegar, maple syrup, and red pepper flakes and set aside.

② In a large skillet over medium heat, heat the oil; add tofu and garlic. Lightly fry 2–3 minutes.

③ Reduce heat to medium-low; add orange juice mixture. Bring to a very low simmer; cook for 7–8 minutes over low heat.

④ In a small bowl, whisk together the cornstarch and water until cornstarch is dissolved. Add to tofu mixture; stir well to combine.

⑤ Bring to a simmer; heat for 3–4 minutes, until sauce thickens. Serve over rice or another whole grain, if desired.

Per Serving
Calories: 219 | Fat: 14g | Sodium: 616mg | Fiber: 1g | Protein: 10g

Saucy Kung Pao Tofu

Try adding in more Asian ingredients to stretch this recipe—bok choy, water chestnuts, or bamboo shoots—and spoon over cooked noodles or rice.

SERVES 6

3 tablespoons soy sauce

2 tablespoons rice vinegar or cooking sherry

1 tablespoon sesame oil

2 (16-ounce) blocks firm or extra-firm tofu, chopped into 1" cubes

1 red bell pepper, chopped

1 green bell pepper, chopped

⅔ cup sliced mushrooms

3 cloves garlic, minced

3 small red or green chili peppers, diced small

1 teaspoon red pepper flakes

2 tablespoons oil

1 teaspoon ginger powder

½ cup water or vegetable broth

½ teaspoon sugar

1½ teaspoons cornstarch

2 scallions, chopped

½ cup peanuts

Folic Acid: 🍎

Vitamin B$_{12}$: NA

Protein: 🍎🍎

Iron: 🍎

Zinc: 🍎🍎

Calcium: 🍎

Vitamin D: very small amounts

1. In a shallow pan or zip-top bag, whisk together the soy sauce, vinegar, and sesame oil. Add tofu; marinate in the refrigerator for at least 1 hour—the longer the better. Drain tofu, reserving marinade.
2. Sauté bell peppers, mushrooms, garlic, chili peppers, and red pepper flakes in oil for 2–3 minutes; add tofu and heat for another 1–2 minutes, until veggies are almost soft.
3. Reduce heat to medium-low; add marinade, ginger powder, water, sugar, and cornstarch, whisking in the cornstarch to avoid lumps.
4. Heat a few more minutes, stirring constantly, until sauce has almost thickened.
5. Add scallions and peanuts; heat for 1 more minute.

Per Serving
Calories: 535 | Fat: 51g | Sodium: 520mg | Fiber: 3g | Protein: 13g

Sesame Baked Tofu

Baking tofu makes it meaty and chewy, and this is a quick and basic marinade to try if you're new to baking tofu. Serve these marinated tofu strips as an entrée or use as a salad topper or as a meat substitute in a sandwich.

SERVES 6

¼ cup soy sauce

2 tablespoons sesame oil

¾ teaspoon garlic powder

½ teaspoon ginger powder

2 (16-ounce) blocks firm or extra-firm tofu, well pressed

Folic Acid: only present in very small amounts

Vitamin B$_{12}$: NA

Protein: 🍎 🍎

Iron: 🍎

Zinc: 🍎

Calcium: 🍎

Vitamin D: NA

1. Whisk together the soy sauce, sesame oil, garlic, and ginger powder; transfer to a wide, shallow pan.
2. Slice the tofu into ½"-thick strips or triangles.
3. Place the tofu in the marinade and coat well. Allow to marinate in the refrigerator for at least 1 hour or overnight.
4. Preheat oven to 400°F.
5. Coat a baking sheet well with nonstick spray or olive oil, or line with foil. Place tofu on sheet.
6. Bake for 20–25 minutes; turn over and bake for another 10–15 minutes, or until done.

Per Serving
Calories: 99 | Fat: 7g | Sodium: 314mg | Fiber: 1g | Protein: 9g

Marinating Tofu

For marinated baked tofu dishes, a zip-top bag can be helpful in getting the tofu well covered with marinade. Place the tofu in the bag, pour the marinade in, seal, and set in the fridge, occasionally turning and lightly shaking to coat all sides of the tofu.

Tofu "Fish" Sticks

Adding seaweed and lemon juice to baked and breaded tofu gives it a "fishy" taste. Crumbled nori sushi sheets would work well too if you can't find kelp or dulse flakes. You could also pan fry these fish sticks in a bit of oil instead of baking, if you prefer.

SERVES 3

½ cup flour

⅓ cup plain or unsweetened fortified soymilk

2 tablespoons lemon juice

1½ cups fine-ground bread crumbs

2 tablespoons kelp or dulse seaweed flakes

1 tablespoon Old Bay seasoning blend

1 teaspoon onion powder

1 (16-ounce) block extra-firm tofu, well pressed

Folic Acid: 🍎🍎
Vitamin B$_{12}$: 🍎🍎
Protein: 🍎🍎🍎
Iron: 🍎🍎
Zinc: 🍎🍎
Calcium: 🍎🍎
Vitamin D: 🍎

1. Preheat oven to 350°F.
2. Place flour in a shallow bowl or pie tin and set aside.
3. Combine the soymilk and lemon juice in a separate shallow bowl or pie tin.
4. In a third bowl or pie tin, combine the bread crumbs, kelp, Old Bay, and onion powder.
5. Slice tofu into twelve, ½"-thick strips. Place each strip into the flour mixture to coat well, then dip into the soymilk. Next, place each strip into the bread crumbs, gently patting to coat well.
6. Bake for 15–20 minutes; turn and bake for another 10–15 minutes, or until crispy. Serve with ketchup or vegan tartar sauce.

Per Serving
Calories: 341 | Fat: 6g | Sodium: 1,070mg | Fiber: 3g | Protein: 19g

Tartar Sauce

To make a simple vegan tartar sauce, combine vegan mayonnaise with sweet pickle relish and a generous squeeze of lemon juice. Or dip your fishy tofu sticks in ketchup or barbecue sauce.

No Shepherd, No Sheep Pie

Sheepless—and shepherdless—pie is a hearty vegan entrée! It's perfect for those nights where you're craving comfort food.

SERVES 6

1½ cups TVP

1½ cups hot water or vegetable broth

2 tablespoons olive oil

½ onion, chopped

2 cloves garlic, minced

1 large carrot, sliced thin

¾ cup sliced mushrooms

½ cup green peas, fresh or frozen, thawed

½ cup vegetable broth

½ cup plus 3 tablespoons soymilk

1 tablespoon flour

5 medium potatoes, cooked

2 tablespoons vegan margarine

¼ teaspoon rosemary

¼ teaspoon sage

½ teaspoon paprika (optional)

½ teaspoon salt, or to taste

¼ teaspoon black pepper

Folic Acid: 🍎

Vitamin B$_{12}$: 🍎🍎

Protein: 🍎🍎🍎

Iron: 🍎

Zinc: 🍎

Calcium: 🍎

Vitamin D: 🍎

1. Preheat oven to 350°F.
2. Combine TVP with hot water and allow to sit for 6–7 minutes. Gently drain any excess moisture.
3. In a large skillet, heat oil and sauté onions, garlic, and carrots until onions are soft, about 5 minutes.
4. Add mushrooms, peas, broth, and ½ cup soymilk. Whisk in flour just until sauce thickens; transfer to a casserole dish.
5. Mash together the potatoes, margarine, 3 tablespoons soymilk, rosemary, sage, paprika, salt, and pepper; spread over the vegetables.
6. Bake for 30–35 minutes, or until lightly browned on top.

Per Serving
Calories: 273 | Fat: 4g | Sodium: 373mg | Fiber: 9g | Protein: 17g

Super-Meaty TVP Meatloaf

With a pinkish hue and chewy texture, this meatloaf impersonates the real thing well. Top with gravy for a Thanksgiving entrée.

SERVES 6

2 cups TVP

1¾ cups hot vegetable broth

1 onion, diced

1 tablespoon oil

¼ cup ketchup

⅓ cup plus 3 tablespoons vegan barbecue sauce

1 cup vital wheat gluten flour

1 cup bread crumbs

1 teaspoon parsley

½ teaspoon sage

½ teaspoon salt, or to taste

¼ teaspoon pepper

Folic Acid: 🍎

Vitamin B$_{12}$: 🍎

Protein: 🍎🍎🍎

Iron: 🍎

Zinc: 🍎

Calcium: 🍎

Vitamin D: NA

① Combine TVP with broth and allow to sit for 6–7 minutes, until rehydrated. Gently squeeze out any excess moisture.

② Sauté onion in oil until translucent, about 3–4 minutes.

③ Preheat oven to 400°F.

④ In a large bowl, combine TVP, onions, ketchup, and ⅓ cup barbecue sauce. Add flour, bread crumbs, and spices.

⑤ Gently press mixture into a lightly greased loaf pan. Drizzle 3 tablespoons of barbecue sauce on top.

⑥ Bake for 45–50 minutes, until lightly browned. Allow to cool for at least 10 minutes before serving, as loaf will set as it cools.

Per Serving
Calories: 321 | Fat: 4g | Sodium: 967mg | Fiber: 7g | Protein: 33g

Sweet and Sour Tempeh

With maple syrup instead of white sugar, this is a sweet and sour that's slightly less sweet than other versions. There's plenty of sauce, so plan on serving with some plain brown rice or another grain to mop it all up.

SERVES 4

1 cup vegetable broth

2 tablespoons soy sauce

1 (8-ounce) package tempeh, diced into cubes

2 tablespoons vegan barbecue sauce

½ teaspoon ground ginger

2 tablespoons maple syrup

⅓ cup rice vinegar or apple cider vinegar

1 tablespoon cornstarch

1 (15-ounce) can pineapple chunks, drained, juice reserved

2 tablespoons olive oil

1 green bell pepper, chopped

1 red bell pepper, chopped

1 yellow onion, chopped

Folic Acid: 🍎

Vitamin B₁₂: NA

Protein: 🍎🍎

Iron: 🍎

Zinc: 🍎🍎

Calcium: 🍎🍎

Vitamin D: NA

① Whisk together the broth and soy sauce and bring to a simmer in a large skillet. Add the tempeh and simmer for 10 minutes. Remove tempeh from the pan; reserve ½ cup broth.

② In a small bowl, whisk together the barbecue sauce, ginger, maple syrup, vinegar, cornstarch, and juice from pineapples until cornstarch is dissolved. Set aside.

③ Heat olive oil in skillet; add tempeh, bell peppers, and onions. Sauté for 1–2 minutes; add sauce mixture and bring to a simmer.

④ Allow to cook until sauce thickens, about 6–8 minutes. Reduce heat and stir in pineapples. Serve over brown rice or another whole grain.

Per Serving
Calories: 325 | Fat: 13g | Sodium: 795mg | Fiber: 2g | Protein: 13g

Italian Balsamic Baked Tofu

A sweet and crunchy Italian-inspired baked tofu delicious on its own or in salads or pastas. The extra marinade makes a great salad dressing!

SERVES 3

1 tablespoon soy sauce

½ teaspoon sugar

¼ cup balsamic vinegar

½ teaspoon garlic powder

2 tablespoons olive oil

½ teaspoon parsley

½ teaspoon basil

¼ teaspoon thyme or oregano

¼ teaspoon salt

¼ teaspoon black pepper

2 (16-ounce) blocks firm or extra-firm tofu, well pressed

Folic Acid: only present in very small amounts

Vitamin B$_{12}$: NA

Protein: 🍎🍎🍎

Iron: 🍎🍎

Zinc: 🍎

Calcium: 🍎

Vitamin D: NA

1. Whisk together all ingredients except tofu and transfer to a wide, shallow pan or Ziploc bag.
2. Slice the tofu into ½"-thick strips or triangles.
3. Place the tofu in the marinade and coat well. Allow to marinate for at least 1 hour or overnight, making sure tofu is well coated in marinade.
4. Preheat oven to 400°F. Coat a baking sheet well with nonstick spray or olive oil, or line with foil. Place tofu on sheet.
5. Bake for 15–20 minutes, turn over, then bake for another 5–10 minutes or until done.

Per Serving
Calories: 255 | Fat: 18g | Sodium: 250mg | Fiber: 2g | Protein: 18g

Agave Mustard Glazed Tofu

Miss honey mustard–glazed ham? Try this vegan version with agave and tofu.

SERVES 3

2 tablespoons lemon juice

2 tablespoons water

1 teaspoon soy sauce

¼ cup agave nectar

2 tablespoons prepared mustard

½ teaspoon garlic powder

½ teaspoon sugar

¾ teaspoon curry powder (optional)

1 (16-ounce) block firm or extra-firm tofu, chopped into 1" cubes

Folic Acid: only present in very small amounts

Vitamin B$_{12}$: NA

Protein: 🍎🍎

Iron: 🍎

Zinc: 🍎

Calcium: 🍎

Vitamin D: NA

1. Whisk together all ingredients in a shallow pan and add tofu. Allow to marinate for at least 1 hour, flipping tofu and basting with sauce.
2. Preheat oven to 400°F.
3. Transfer tofu to a baking sheet or casserole dish, basting with extra sauce. Bake tofu for 20–25 minutes, turning over once and spooning extra marinade over the top.

Per Serving
Calories: 174 | Fat: 4g | Sodium: 259mg | Fiber: 1g | Protein: 10g

Spicy Chili Basil Tofu

This saucy stir-fry is a favorite in Thailand when made with chicken and fish sauce, but many restaurants offer a vegetarian version with soy sauce and tofu instead. Serve with rice or rice noodles to sop up all the sauce.

SERVES 3

4 cloves garlic, minced

5 small red or green chilies, diced

3 shallots, diced

2 tablespoons oil

1 (16-ounce) block firm tofu, diced

¼ cup soy sauce

1 tablespoon vegetarian oyster mushroom sauce

1 teaspoon sugar

1 bunch Thai or holy basil leaves, whole

Folic Acid: 🍎

Vitamin B₁₂: NA

Protein: 🍎🍎

Iron: 🍎

Zinc: 🍎

Calcium: 🍎

Vitamin D: NA

1. In a large skillet, sauté garlic, chilies, and shallots in oil until fragrant and browned, about 3–4 minutes.
2. Add tofu and heat for another 2–3 minutes until tofu is just lightly golden brown.
3. Reduce heat to medium-low and add soy sauce, mushroom sauce, and sugar, whisking to combine and dissolve sugar. Heat 2–3 more minutes, stirring frequently, then add basil and heat, stirring 1 more minute, just until basil is wilted.

Per Serving
Calories: 207 | Fat: 13g | Sodium: 1,414mg | Fiber: 1g | Protein: 12g

Make It Last

If tofu and chilies aren't enough for you, add in some onions, mushrooms, or green bell peppers to fill it out. Or, for a bit of variety, try it with half basil and half fresh mint leaves.

Chili and Curry Baked Tofu

If you like tofu and you like Indian- or Thai-style curries, you'll love this spicy baked tofu, which tastes like a slowly simmered curry in each bite. Use the extra marinade to dress a bowl of plain steamed rice.

SERVES 3

⅓ cup coconut milk

½ teaspoon garlic powder

1 teaspoon cumin

1 teaspoon curry powder

½ teaspoon turmeric

2–3 small chilies, minced

2 tablespoons maple syrup

1 (16-ounce) block firm or extra-firm tofu, sliced into thin strips

Folic Acid: only present in very small amounts

Vitamin B$_{12}$: NA

Protein: 🍎 🍎

Iron: 🍎 🍎

Zinc: 🍎

Calcium: 🍎

Vitamin D: NA

1. Whisk together coconut milk, garlic powder, cumin, curry, turmeric, chilies, and maple syrup in a shallow bowl. Add tofu and marinate for at least 1 hour, flipping once or twice to coat well.
2. Preheat oven to 425°F.
3. Transfer tofu to a casserole dish in a single layer, reserving marinade.
4. Bake for 8–10 minutes. Turn tofu over, and spoon 1–2 tablespoons of marinade over the tofu. Bake 10–12 more minutes.

Per Serving
Calories: 178 | Fat: 9g | Sodium: 54mg | Fiber: 1g | Protein: 10g

Nutty Pesto-Crusted Tofu

Make sure the coating is completely dry before trying these crispy, herbed tofu cutlets.

SERVES 6

½ cup roasted cashews

½ cup basil, packed

3 cloves garlic

½ cup nutritional yeast

⅔ cup bread crumbs

½ teaspoon salt

¼ teaspoon pepper

⅔ cup flour

⅔ cup fortified soymilk

2 (16-ounce) blocks firm or extra-firm tofu, pressed

Oil for pan frying (optional)

Folic Acid: 🍎🍎🍎

Vitamin B₁₂: 🍎🍎🍎 Includes 100% of the DRI

Protein: 🍎🍎🍎

Iron: 🍎🍎

Zinc: 🍎🍎🍎

Calcium: 🍎🍎

Vitamin D: 🍎

1. Preheat oven to 350°F. In a blender or food processor, process the nuts until coarse and fine but not powdery. Separately, process the basil and garlic until finely minced.
2. Combine the cashews, basil, garlic, nutritional yeast, bread crumbs, salt, and pepper in a bowl. Place the flour in a separate shallow bowl and the soymilk in a third bowl.
3. Slice each block of tofu into triangular cutlets, about ¾"-thick. Using tongs, dip in flour and coat well, then dip in soymilk. Next, coat well with the basil and bread crumb mixture and transfer to a lightly greased baking sheet.
4. Bake for 10–12 minutes, or until lightly crispy. Alternatively, tofu can be pan fried in oil over medium heat for a few minutes on each side until lightly crispy

Per Serving
Calories: 275 | Fat: 10g | Sodium: 376mg | Fiber: 3g | Protein: 17g

Easy Lemon Thyme Marinated Tofu

The leftover marinade can be whisked with some extra olive oil for a lemony salad dressing.

SERVES 3

3 tablespoons lemon juice

3 tablespoons soy sauce

1 tablespoon olive oil

3 tablespoons water

1 tablespoon chopped fresh or 2 teaspoons dried thyme

1 (16-ounce) block firm or extra-firm tofu, pressed

Dash salt and pepper

Folic Acid: only present in small amounts

Vitamin B$_{12}$: NA

Protein: 🍎 🍎

Iron: 🍎

Zinc: 🍎

Calcium: 🍎

Vitamin D: NA

① In a shallow pan, whisk together the lemon juice, soy sauce, olive oil, water, and thyme.

② Slice pressed tofu into desired shape, about ½"-thick, and cover with marinade. Allow to marinate for at least 1 hour, preferably longer.

③ Preheat oven to 400°F and transfer tofu to a lightly greased baking sheet or casserole dish. Sprinkle with a bit of salt and pepper.

④ Bake tofu for 10–12 minutes or until lightly crispy.

Per Serving
Calories: 110 | Fat: 6g | Sodium: 498mg | Fiber: 0g | Protein: 10g

Five-Spice Glazed Tofu

Chinese five-spice is a blend of spices with an exotic and unique taste. Everyone will be asking you what it is!

SERVES 3

1 (16-ounce) block firm tofu, well pressed

½ cup water

2 tablespoons soy sauce

1 tablespoon sesame oil

1 tablespoon brown sugar

2 cloves garlic, minced

¾ teaspoon Chinese five-spice

Folic Acid: only present in very small amounts

Vitamin B$_{12}$: NA

Protein:

Iron:

Zinc:

Calcium:

Vitamin D: NA

1. Slice tofu into ½"-thick slabs or triangles.
2. Whisk together the water, soy sauce, sesame oil, brown sugar, garlic, and five-spice in a shallow pan, and add tofu, covering well. Allow to marinate for at least 30 minutes.
3. Preheat oven to 350°F. Transfer tofu and marinade to a baking sheet or casserole dish and bake for 10–15 minutes on each side.

Per Serving
Calories: 142 | Fat: 8g | Sodium: 651mg | Fiber: 0g | Protein: 10g

CHAPTER 6

Sides

Coconut Rice

Serve coconut rice as a simple side dish or pair it with spicy Thai and Indian curries or stir-fries.

SERVES 6

1 cup water

1 (14-ounce) can coconut milk

1½ cups white rice, uncooked

⅓ cup coconut flakes

1 teaspoon lime juice

½ teaspoon salt, or to taste

Folic Acid: 🍎🍎

Vitamin B$_{12}$: NA

Protein: 🍎

Iron: 🍎🍎

Zinc: 🍎

Calcium: 🍎

Vitamin D: NA

1. In a large pot, combine the water, coconut milk, and rice; bring to a simmer. Cover, and allow to cook 20 minutes, or until rice is done.
2. In a separate skillet, toast the coconut flakes over low heat until lightly golden, about 3 minutes. Gently stir constantly to avoid burning.
3. Combine coconut flakes with cooked rice; stir in lime juice and salt.

Per Serving
Calories: 320 | Fat: 16g | Sodium: 207mg | Fiber: 1g | Protein: 5g

Greek Lemon Rice with Spinach

Greek "spanakorizo" is seasoned with fresh lemon, herbs, and black pepper. Serve with Lemon Basil Tofu (see recipe in Chapter 5) for a citrusy meal.

SERVES 4

1 onion, chopped

4 cloves garlic, minced

2 tablespoons olive oil

¾ cup white rice, uncooked

1½ cups water or vegetable broth

1 (6-ounce) can tomato paste

2 bunches fresh spinach, trimmed

2 tablespoons chopped fresh parsley

1 tablespoon chopped fresh mint or dill (optional)

2 tablespoons lemon juice

½ teaspoon salt, or to taste

½ teaspoon fresh ground black pepper

Folic Acid: 🍎🍎🍎

Vitamin B$_{12}$: NA

Protein: 🍎🍎

Iron: 🍎🍎🍎

Zinc: 🍎🍎

Calcium: 🍎🍎🍎

Vitamin D: NA

1. Sauté onions and garlic in olive oil for 1–2 minutes; add rice, stirring to lightly toast.
2. Add water; cover, and heat for 10–12 minutes.
3. Add tomato paste, spinach, and parsley. Cover, and cook for another 5 minutes, or until spinach is wilted and rice is cooked.
4. Stir in fresh mint, lemon juice, salt, and pepper.

Per Serving
Calories: 295 | Fat: 8g | Sodium: 488mg | Fiber: 7g | Protein: 10g

Italian Rice Salad

Double this marinated rice salad recipe for a potluck, picnic, or baby shower.

SERVES 8

⅓ cup red wine vinegar

1 tablespoon balsamic vinegar

2 teaspoons Dijon mustard

½ cup olive oil

4 cloves garlic, minced

1 teaspoon basil

⅓ cup chopped fresh parsley

2 cups cooked rice

1 cup green peas, fresh or frozen, thawed

1 carrot, grated

½ cup roasted red peppers, chopped

½ cup green olives, sliced

Salt and pepper, to taste

Folic Acid: 🍎

Vitamin B$_{12}$: NA

Protein: 🍎

Iron: 🍎

Zinc: 🍎

Calcium: 🍎

Vitamin D: NA

① Whisk or shake together the vinegars, mustard, olive oil, garlic, basil, and parsley.

② In a large bowl, combine rice with remaining ingredients except salt and pepper. Toss with dressing mixture; coat well.

③ Taste, and season with salt and pepper, to taste.

④ Chill for at least 30 minutes before serving to allow flavors to meld. Gently toss again just before serving.

Per Serving
Calories: 219 | Fat: 16g | Sodium: 302mg | Fiber: 2g | Protein: 2g

Pineapple Lime Rice

Instead of pineapple, fresh cubed mango would also add a sweet flavor to this simple zesty side.

SERVES 4

2 cups warm, cooked brown or white rice

2 tablespoons vegan margarine

1½ tablespoons lime juice

⅓ cup chopped fresh cilantro

1 (16-ounce) can pineapple tidbits, drained

Dash salt

Folic Acid: 🍎

Vitamin B$_{12}$: NA

Protein: 🍎

Iron: 🍎

Zinc: 🍎

Calcium: 🍎

Vitamin D: NA

1. Stir margarine into hot rice until melted and combined.
2. Add remaining ingredients; toss gently to combine. Taste, and add a dash of salt, to taste.

Per Serving
Calories: 222 | Fat: 6g | Sodium: 83mg | Fiber: 2g | Protein: 3g

Sesame Snow Pea Rice Pilaf

The leftovers from this rice pilaf can be enjoyed chilled the next day as a cold rice salad.

SERVES 8

4 cups cooked rice

2 tablespoons olive oil

1 tablespoon sesame oil

2 tablespoons soy sauce

3 tablespoons apple cider vinegar

1 teaspoon sugar

1 cup snow peas, chopped

¾ cup baby corn, chopped

3 scallions, chopped

2 tablespoons chopped fresh parsley

½ teaspoon sea salt

Folic Acid: 🌶🌶

Vitamin B$_{12}$: NA

Protein: 🌶

Iron: 🌶

Zinc: 🌶

Calcium: 🌶

Vitamin D: NA

1. In a large pot over low heat, combine the rice, olive oil, sesame oil, soy sauce, vinegar, and sugar, stirring well to combine.
2. Add snow peas, baby corn, and scallions and heat until warmed through and vegetables are lightly cooked, stirring frequently, so the rice doesn't burn.
3. While still hot, stir in fresh parsley and season well with sea salt.

Per Serving
Calories: 172 | Fat: 5g | Sodium: 420mg | Fiber: 1g | Protein: 3g

Baked Millet Patties

Serve these nutty whole-grain patties topped with Mango Citrus Salsa (see recipe in Chapter 4), Goddess Dressing (see recipe in Chapter 7), or another dressing or sauce.

YIELDS 8 PATTIES

1½ cups cooked millet

½ cup tahini

1 cup bread crumbs

1 teaspoon parsley

¾ teaspoon garlic powder

½ teaspoon onion powder (optional)

⅓ teaspoon salt, or to taste

Folic Acid: 🍎🍎

Vitamin B$_{12}$: NA

Protein: 🍎🍎

Iron: 🍎🍎

Zinc: 🍎🍎

Calcium: 🍎

Vitamin D: NA

① Preheat oven to 350°F.

② Combine all ingredients together in a bowl; mash to mix well.

③ Use your hands to press firmly into patties, about 1" thick. Place on a baking sheet.

④ Bake for 10–12 minutes on each side.

Per Patty
Calories: 285 | Fat: 10g | Sodium: 214mg | Fiber: 5g | Protein: 9g

Fruited Fall Quinoa

Cranberries and apricots make a sweet combo; add some sage and thyme to give it some more warming flavors and it would make an excellent Thanksgiving side dish.

SERVES 4

1 cup quinoa

2 cups apple juice

1 cup water

½ onion, diced

2 ribs celery, diced

2 tablespoons vegan margarine

½ teaspoon nutmeg

½ teaspoon cinnamon

¼ teaspoon cloves

½ cup dried cranberries

½ cup dried apricots, chopped

1 teaspoon parsley

¼ teaspoon salt, or to taste

Folic Acid:

Vitamin B$_{12}$: NA

Protein:

Iron:

Zinc:

Calcium:

Vitamin D: NA

① In a large pot, combine quinoa, apple juice, and water. Cover, and simmer for 15 minutes, or until done.

② In a large skillet, heat onion and celery in margarine, stirring frequently, until soft, about 5 minutes.

③ Over low heat, combine onions and celery with quinoa; add remaining ingredients, tossing gently to combine. Heat for 3–4 more minutes.

Per Serving
Calories: 360 | Fat: 9g | Sodium: 252mg | Fiber: 6g | Protein: 7g

Lemon Cilantro Couscous

This flavorful couscous is a light and easy side dish, or top it off with a vegetable stew or some stir-fried or roasted veggies for an entrée.

SERVES 4

2 cups vegetable broth

1 cup couscous

⅓ cup lemon juice

½ cup chopped fresh cilantro

¼ teaspoon salt, or to taste

Folic Acid: 🍎

Vitamin B$_{12}$: NA

Protein: 🍎

Iron: 🍎

Zinc: 🍎

Calcium: only present in very small amounts

Vitamin D: NA

1. Bring broth to a simmer; add couscous. Turn off heat; cover, and let stand for 10 minutes, until soft. Fluff with a fork.
2. Stir in lemon juice and cilantro; season with salt, to taste.

Per Serving
Calories: 174 | Fat: 0g | Sodium: 621mg | Fiber: 2g | Protein: 6g

What Is Couscous?

Couscous isn't technically a whole grain, but rather whole-wheat semolina pasta. But its small size and grainy texture gives it more in common with whole grains than pasta.

Lemon Quinoa Veggie Salad

If you prefer to use fresh veggies, any kind will do. Steamed broccoli or fresh tomatoes would work well.

SERVES 4

4 cups vegetable broth

1½ cups quinoa

1 cup frozen mixed veggies, thawed

¼ cup lemon juice

¼ cup olive oil

1 teaspoon garlic powder

½ teaspoon salt

¼ teaspoon black pepper

2 tablespoons chopped fresh cilantro or parsley (optional)

Folic Acid: 🍎🍎🍎

Vitamin B$_{12}$: NA

Protein: 🍎🍎

Iron: 🍎🍎

Zinc: 🍎🍎🍎

Calcium: 🍎

Vitamin D: NA

1. In a large pot, bring broth to a boil. Add quinoa; cover, and simmer for 15–20 minutes, stirring occasionally, until liquid is absorbed and quinoa is cooked.
2. Add mixed veggies; stir to combine.
3. Remove from heat; combine with remaining ingredients. Serve hot or cold.

Per Serving
Calories: 408 | Fat: 18g | Sodium: 1,261mg | Fiber: 7g | Protein: 11g

Mediterranean Quinoa Pilaf

Bring this vibrant whole-grain dish, inspired by the flavors of the Mediterranean, to a vegan potluck and watch it magically disappear.

SERVES 6

1½ cups quinoa

3 cups vegetable broth

3 tablespoons balsamic vinegar

2 tablespoons olive oil

1 tablespoon lemon juice

⅓ teaspoon salt, or to taste

½ cup sun-dried tomatoes, chopped

½ cup artichoke hearts, chopped

½ cup black or kalamata olives, sliced

Folic Acid: 🍎🍎

Vitamin B₁₂: NA

Protein: 🍎

Iron: 🍎🍎

Zinc: 🍎🍎

Calcium: 🍎

Vitamin D: NA

1. In a large skillet or saucepan, bring the quinoa and broth to a boil; reduce to a simmer. Cover, and allow quinoa to cook until liquid is absorbed, about 15 minutes. Remove from heat, fluff quinoa with a fork, and allow to stand another 5 minutes.
2. Stir in the vinegar, olive oil, lemon juice, and salt; add remaining ingredients, gently tossing to combine. Serve hot.

Per Serving
Calories: 348 | Fat: 21g | Sodium: 778mg | Fiber: 4g | Protein: 7g

Millet and Butternut Squash Casserole

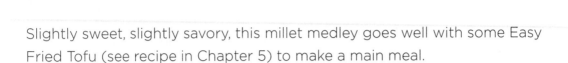

Slightly sweet, slightly savory, this millet medley goes well with some Easy Fried Tofu (see recipe in Chapter 5) to make a main meal.

SERVES 4

1 cup millet

2 cups vegetable broth

1 small butternut squash, peeled, seeded, and chopped

½ cup water

1 teaspoon curry powder

½ cup orange juice

2 tablespoons nutritional yeast

½ teaspoon sea salt, or to taste

Folic Acid: 🍎🍎🍎

Vitamin B$_{12}$: 🍎🍎🍎

Protein: 🍎

Iron: 🍎

Zinc: 🍎

Calcium: 🍎

Vitamin D: NA

1. In a small pot, cook millet in broth until done, about 20–30 minutes.
2. In a separate pan, heat butternut squash in water. Cover, and allow to cook for 10–15 minutes, until squash is almost soft. Remove lid and drain extra water.
3. Combine millet with squash over low heat; add curry and orange juice, stirring to combine well.
4. Heat for 3–4 more minutes; add nutritional yeast and season with salt.

Per Serving
Calories: 242 | Fat: 2g | Sodium: 767mg | Fiber: 6g | Protein: 7g

Orange and Raisin Curried Couscous

This is another whole-grain salad or pilaf that can be served either hot or cold. Cranberries, currants, or dates may be used instead of raisins.

SERVES 6

2 cups water or vegetable broth

1½ cups couscous

½ cup orange juice

1 onion, chopped

2 tablespoons olive oil

½ teaspoon coriander powder

1 teaspoon curry powder

2 scallions, chopped

¾ cup golden raisins

¾ cup sliced almonds or pine nuts

Folic Acid: 🌶

Vitamin B$_{12}$: NA

Protein: 🌶🌶

Iron: 🌶

Zinc: 🌶

Calcium: 🌶

Vitamin D: NA

1. Bring water to a boil; add couscous and remove from heat.
2. Stir in orange juice; cover, and allow to sit for 15 minutes, until most of the liquid is absorbed and couscous is soft.
3. Heat onion in olive oil for 1–2 minutes; add spices and heat for 1 more minute, until fragrant.
4. Combine couscous with spices; add scallions, raisins, and nuts.

Per Serving
Calories: 520 | Fat: 16g | Sodium: 483mg | Fiber: 7g | Protein: 14g

Mexican Rice with Corn and Peppers

Although Mexican rice is usually just a filling for burritos or served as a side dish, this recipe loads up the veggies, making it hearty enough for a main dish. Use frozen or canned veggies if you need to save time.

SERVES 4

2 cloves garlic, minced

1 cup white rice, uncooked

2 tablespoons olive oil

2 cups vegetable broth

1 cup tomato paste or 4 large tomatoes, puréed

1 green bell pepper, chopped

1 red bell pepper, chopped

Kernels from 1 ear of corn

1 carrot, diced

1 teaspoon chili powder

½ teaspoon cumin

⅓ teaspoon oregano

⅓ teaspoon cayenne pepper, or to taste

⅓ teaspoon salt, or to taste

Folic Acid: 🍎🍎🍎

Vitamin B$_{12}$: NA

Protein: 🍎🍎

Iron: 🍎🍎🍎

Zinc: 🍎

Calcium: 🍎

Vitamin D: NA

1. In a large skillet over medium-high heat, add garlic, rice, and olive oil. Toast the rice, stirring frequently, until just golden brown, about 2–3 minutes.
2. Reduce heat; add broth and remaining ingredients.
3. Bring to a simmer; cover, and allow to cook until liquid is absorbed and rice is cooked, about 20–25 minutes, stirring occasionally.
4. Adjust seasonings to taste.

Per Serving
Calories: 342 | Fat: 8g | Sodium: 1,442mg | Fiber: 6g | Protein: 8g

Vegan Burritos

Brown some vegetarian chorizo or mock sausage crumbles, mix with Mexican Rice with Corn and Peppers, and wrap in tortillas, perhaps topped with some shredded vegan cheese, to make vegan burritos.

Spicy Southern Jambalaya

Make this spicy and smoky Southern rice dish a main meal by adding in some browned mock sausage or sautéed tofu.

SERVES 6

2 tablespoons olive oil

1 onion, chopped

1 bell pepper, any color, chopped

1 rib celery, diced

1 (14-ounce) can diced tomatoes, undrained

3 cups water or vegetable broth

2 cups white rice, uncooked

1 bay leaf

1 teaspoon paprika

½ teaspoon thyme

½ teaspoon oregano

½ teaspoon garlic powder

1 cup corn or thawed, frozen mixed diced veggies (optional)

½ teaspoon cayenne or hot Tabasco sauce, to taste

Folic Acid: 🍎

Vitamin B$_{12}$: NA

Protein: 🍎

Iron: 🍎

Zinc: 🍎🍎

Calcium: 🍎

Vitamin D: NA

1. In a large skillet or stockpot, heat olive oil. Sauté onion, bell pepper, and celery until almost soft, about 3 minutes.
2. Reduce heat and add remaining ingredients except veggies and cayenne; cover. Bring to a low simmer; cook for 20 minutes, until rice is done, stirring occasionally.
3. Add veggies and cayenne; cook just until heated through, about 3 minutes. Adjust seasonings to taste. Remove bay leaf before serving.

Per Serving
Calories: 304 | Fat: 7g | Sodium: 100mg | Fiber: 4g | Protein: 7g

Got Leftovers?

Heat up some refried beans and wrap up your leftover jambalaya in tortillas with some salsa and shredded lettuce to make New Orleans-style vegetable burritos!

Sun-Dried Tomato Risotto with Spinach and Pine Nuts

The tomatoes carry the flavor in this easy risotto—no butter, cheese, or wine (not like that's on the menu now anyway!) is needed. But if you're a gourmand who keeps truffle, hazelnut, pine nut, or another gourmet oil on hand, now's the time to use it, instead of the margarine.

SERVES 6

1 yellow onion, diced

4 cloves garlic, minced

2 tablespoons olive oil

1½ cups Arborio rice, uncooked

5–6 cups vegetable broth

⅔ cup rehydrated sun-dried tomatoes, sliced

½ cup fresh spinach

1 tablespoon chopped fresh basil (optional)

2 tablespoons vegan margarine (optional)

2 tablespoons nutritional yeast

Salt and pepper, to taste

¼ cup pine nuts

Folic Acid: 🍎🍎🍎

Vitamin B$_{12}$: 🍎🍎🍎

Protein: 🍎

Iron: 🍎🍎

Zinc: 🍎🍎

Calcium: only present in very small amounts

Vitamin D: NA

1. Heat onion and garlic in olive oil until just soft, about 2–3 minutes. Add rice; toast for 1 minute, stirring constantly.
2. Add ¾ cup broth; stir to combine. When most of the liquid has been absorbed, add another ½ cup, stirring constantly. Continue adding liquid ½ cup at a time until rice is cooked, about 20 minutes.
3. Add another ½ cup broth, tomatoes, spinach, and basil; reduce heat to low. Stir to combine well. Heat for 3–4 minutes, until tomatoes are soft and spinach is wilted.
4. Stir in margarine and nutritional yeast. Taste, then season with salt and pepper, to taste.
5. Allow to cool slightly, then top with pine nuts. Risotto will thicken a bit as it cools.

Per Serving
Calories: 294 | Fat: 9g | Sodium: 882 | Fiber: 3g | Protein: 6g

"Cheesy" Broccoli and Rice Casserole

If you're substituting frozen broccoli, there's no need to cook it first, just thaw and use about 1¼ cups.

SERVES 6

1 head broccoli, chopped small

1 onion, chopped

4 cloves garlic, minced

2 tablespoons olive oil

2 tablespoons flour

2 cups unsweetened soymilk

½ cup vegetable broth

2 tablespoons nutritional yeast

1 tablespoon vegan margarine

¼ teaspoon nutmeg

¼ teaspoon mustard powder

½ teaspoon salt

3½ cups cooked rice

⅔ cup bread crumbs or crushed vegan crackers

Folic Acid: 🍎🍎🍎

Vitamin B$_{12}$: 🍎🍎🍎

Protein: 🍎🍎

Iron: 🍎🍎

Zinc: 🍎🍎

Calcium: 🍎🍎

Vitamin D: 🍎

① Preheat oven to 325°F.

② Steam or microwave broccoli until just barely soft; do not overcook.

③ Sauté onions and garlic in olive oil until soft, about 3–4 minutes. Reduce heat and add flour, stirring continuously to combine.

④ Add soymilk and vegetable broth and heat, stirring, until thickened. Remove from heat and stir in nutritional yeast, margarine, nutmeg, mustard powder, and salt.

⑤ Combine sauce, steamed broccoli, and cooked rice and transfer to a large casserole or baking dish. Sprinkle the top with bread crumbs or vegan crackers.

⑥ Cover and bake for 25 minutes. Uncover and cook for another 10 minutes.

Per Serving
Calories: 318 | Fat: 9g | Sodium: 268mg | Fiber: 5g | Protein: 10g

Barley and Mushroom Pilaf

An earthy-flavored pilaf with mushrooms and nutty toasted barley. This one will really stick to your ribs—or your baby bump!

SERVES 4

1 cup sliced porcini mushrooms

1 cup sliced shiitake mushrooms

2 ribs celery, diced

½ onion, chopped

3 tablespoons vegan margarine or olive oil

1¼ cups barley

3¾ cups vegetable broth

1 bay leaf

¼ teaspoon sage

½ teaspoon parsley

½ teaspoon thyme

Folic Acid: 🍎

Vitamin B₁₂: NA

Protein: 🍎 🍎

Iron: 🍎

Zinc: 🍎 🍎

Calcium: 🍎

Vitamin D: only present in small amounts

1. In a large skillet or stockpot, sauté mushrooms, celery, and onion in 2 tablespoons margarine until almost soft, about 2–3 minutes.
2. Add barley and remaining 1 tablespoon of margarine; allow to toast for 1–2 minutes, stirring frequently.
3. When barley starts to turn brown, add broth and seasonings.
4. Bring to a simmer; cover, and allow to cook for 20–25 minutes, stirring occasionally, until liquid is absorbed and barley is cooked. Remove bay leaf before serving.

Per Serving
Calories: 323 | Fat: 9g | Sodium: 1,025mg | Fiber: 11g | Protein: 8g

Cooking Barley

Be sure you pick up either pearl or quick-cooking barley, and not the hulled variety, which takes ages to cook. Pearl barley is done in 20–25 minutes, and quick-cooking barley is done in about 10, so adjust the cooking times as needed. Barley can also be cooked in your rice steamer with about 2½ cups liquid for each cup of barley.

Bulgur Wheat Tabbouleh Salad with Tomatoes

Though you'll need to adjust the cooking time, of course, you can try this tabbouleh recipe with just about any whole grain. Bulgur wheat is traditional, but quinoa, millet, or amaranth would also work.

SERVES 4

1¼ cups boiling water or vegetable broth

1 cup bulgur wheat

3 tablespoons olive oil

¼ cup lemon juice

1 teaspoon garlic powder

½ teaspoon salt

½ teaspoon pepper

3 scallions, chopped

½ cup chopped fresh mint

½ cup chopped fresh parsley

1 (15-ounce) can chickpeas, drained (optional)

3 large tomatoes, diced

Folic Acid: 🍎

Vitamin B₁₂: NA

Protein: 🍎

Iron: 🍎🍎

Zinc: 🍎🍎

Calcium: 🍎

Vitamin D: NA

1. Pour boiling water over bulgur wheat. Cover; allow to sit for 30 minutes, or until bulgur wheat is soft.
2. Toss bulgur wheat with olive oil, lemon juice, garlic powder, and salt, stirring well to coat. Combine with remaining ingredients, adding in tomatoes last.
3. Allow to chill for at least 1 hour before serving.

Per Serving
Calories: 252 | Fat: 11g | Sodium: 315mg | Fiber: 10g | Protein: 7g

Leftover Tabbouleh Sandwiches

Spread a slice of bread or a tortilla with some hummus, then layer leftover tabbouleh, sweet pickle relish, thinly sliced cucumbers, and some lettuce to make a quick sandwich or wrap for lunch.

Confetti "Rice" with TVP

If you like Mexican rice, try this whole-grain version with barley and TVP.

SERVES 6

2 tablespoons olive oil

1 onion, chopped

2 cloves garlic, minced

1 cup barley

1 (14-ounce) can diced tomatoes

2 cups vegetable broth

1 teaspoon chili powder

½ teaspoon cumin

¾ cup TVP

1 cup hot water or vegetable broth

1 tablespoon soy sauce

1 cup thawed, frozen veggie mix (peas, corn, and carrots)

1 teaspoon parsley

½ teaspoon salt, or to taste

Folic Acid: 🍎

Vitamin B$_{12}$: NA

Protein: 🍎🍎

Iron: 🍎

Zinc: 🍎

Calcium: 🍎

Vitamin D: NA

1. In a large skillet, heat the olive oil. Add the onion and garlic; sauté for 1–2 minutes. Add barley; toast for 1 minute, stirring constantly.
2. Add tomatoes including liquid, broth, chili powder, and cumin. Cook until barley is almost soft, about 15 minutes.
3. While barley is cooking, combine TVP with hot water and soy sauce; allow to sit for 8–10 minutes, until TVP is rehydrated. Drain any excess liquid.
4. When barley is almost done cooking, add rehydrated TVP, veggies, parsley, and salt. Heat for another 5 minutes, or until done.

Per Serving
Calories: 258 | Fat: 5g | Sodium: 628mg | Fiber: 11g | Protein: 12g

Turn It Into Tacos

Use this "meaty" Mexican "rice" as a base for burritos or crunchy tacos instead of meat, along with some shredded lettuce, vegan cheese, and nondairy sour cream or serve alongside some cooked beans for a healthy Mexican meal.

Quinoa and Fresh Herb Stuffing

Substitute dried herbs if you have to, but fresh is best in this untraditional stuffing recipe.

SERVES 6

1 yellow onion, chopped

2 ribs celery, diced

¼ cup vegan margarine

1 teaspoon chopped fresh rosemary

2 teaspoons chopped fresh marjoram

1½ tablespoons chopped fresh thyme

1 tablespoon chopped fresh sage

6 slices dried bread, cubed

1¼ cups vegetable broth

2 cups cooked quinoa

¾ teaspoon salt, or to taste

½ teaspoon pepper

Folic Acid: 🍎

Vitamin B$_{12}$: NA

Protein: 🍎

Iron: 🍎

Zinc: 🍎

Calcium: 🍎

Vitamin D: NA

1. Preheat oven to 400°F.
2. Sauté onion and celery in margarine until soft, about 6–8 minutes. Add fresh herbs; heat for another minute, just until fragrant.
3. Remove from heat; pour into a casserole dish.
4. Add bread; combine well. Add vegetable broth to moisten bread; you may need a bit more or less than 1¼ cups.
5. Add cooked quinoa, salt, and pepper; combine well.
6. Cover; bake for 30 minutes.

Per Serving
Calories: 220 | Fat: 10g | Sodium: 739mg | Fiber: 3g | Protein: 5g

Stuffed-Up Stuffing

Stuffing works best with dried bread to better absorb all that flavor and moisture. Leave your bread out for a couple days, or lightly toast in a 275°F oven for 20 minutes on each side. For a more textured stuffing, add in ¾ cup chopped dried apricots, or ¾ cup chopped nuts (walnuts, cashews, or pecans), or sauté some mushrooms or a grated carrot along with the onions and celery.

Summer Squash and Barley Risotto

A smooth and saucy risotto with barley instead of rice is perfect for those hot summer nights—or those pregnancy hot flashes. Fresh asparagus instead of squash would also be lovely in this untraditional risotto. Top it off with some vegan Parmesan cheese, if you happen to have some on hand.

SERVES 4

4 cloves garlic, minced

½ onion, diced

1 zucchini, chopped

1 yellow squash, chopped

2 tablespoons olive oil

1 cup pearled barley

3–4 cups vegetable broth

2 tablespoons chopped fresh basil

2 tablespoons nutritional yeast

2 tablespoons vegan margarine

Salt and pepper, to taste

Folic Acid: 🍎🍎🍎

Vitamin B$_{12}$: 🍎🍎🍎

Protein: 🍎

Iron: 🍎

Zinc: 🍎🍎

Calcium: 🍎

Vitamin D: NA

1. Sauté garlic, onions, zucchini, and yellow squash in olive oil until soft, about 3–4 minutes. Add barley; heat for 1 minute, stirring to coat well with oil and to prevent burning.
2. Add 1 cup broth; bring to a simmer. Cover; allow to cook for a few minutes, until broth is almost absorbed.
3. Add another cup of broth; continue cooking until barley is soft, about 20–25 minutes, adding more broth as needed.
4. When barley is done, add an additional ¼ cup broth and basil; stir well to combine just until heated through.
5. Stir in yeast and margarine; season generously with salt and pepper, to taste.

Per Serving
Calories: 323 | Fat: 13g | Sodium: 797mg | Fiber: 9g | Protein: 7g

Indian-Spiced Chickpeas with Spinach (Chana Masala)

This is a mild recipe, suitable for the whole family, but if you want to turn up the heat, toss in some fresh minced chilies or a hearty dash of cayenne pepper. It's enjoyable as is for a side dish or piled on top of rice or another grain for a main meal.

SERVES 3

1 onion, chopped

2 cloves garlic, minced

2 tablespoons vegan margarine

¾ teaspoon coriander

1 teaspoon cumin

1 (15-ounce) can chickpeas, undrained

3 tomatoes, puréed or ⅔ cup tomato paste

½ teaspoon curry

¼ teaspoon turmeric

¼ teaspoon salt

1 tablespoon lemon juice

1 bunch fresh spinach

Folic Acid: 🍎🍎🍎

Vitamin B₁₂: NA

Protein: 🍎🍎

Iron: 🍎🍎🍎

Zinc: 🍎🍎🍎

Calcium: 🍎🍎

Vitamin D: NA

1. In a large skillet, sauté onions and garlic in margarine until almost soft, about 2 minutes.
2. Reduce heat to medium-low and add coriander and cumin. Toast the spices, stirring, for 1 minute.
3. Add the chickpeas with liquid in can, tomatoes, curry, turmeric, and salt and bring to a slow simmer. Allow to cook until most of the liquid has been absorbed, about 10–12 minutes, stirring occasionally, then add lemon juice.
4. Add spinach and stir to combine. Cook just until spinach begins to wilt, about 1 minute. Serve immediately.

Per Serving
Calories: 306 | Fat: 10g | Sodium: 818mg | Fiber: 11g | Protein: 12g

Sesame Soy Asparagus and Mushrooms

Fresh asparagus in season has such a vibrant taste, it needs very little enhancement. If you can't find fresh asparagus, don't bother trying this with the canned variety; it's not the same at all!

SERVES 4

1 pound fresh asparagus, trimmed and chopped

¾ cup chopped mushrooms

2 teaspoons sesame oil

1 teaspoon soy sauce

½ teaspoon sugar

2 tablespoons sesame seeds (optional)

Folic Acid: 🍎🍎

Vitamin B₁₂: NA

Protein: 🍎

Iron: 🍎

Zinc: 🍎

Calcium: 🍎

Vitamin D: only present in very small amounts

1. Preheat oven to 350°F.
2. Place asparagus and mushrooms on a baking pan and roast for 10 minutes.
3. Remove pan from oven; drizzle with sesame oil, soy sauce, and sugar; and toss gently to coat.
4. Roast in oven for 5–6 more minutes.
5. Remove from oven, and toss with sesame seeds.

Per Serving
Calories: 48 | Fat: 2g | Sodium: 77mg | Fiber: 3g | Protein: 3g

Potatoes "Au Gratin" Casserole

You'll never miss the boxed version after trying these easy potatoes!

SERVES 4

4 potatoes

1 onion, chopped

1 tablespoon vegan margarine

2 tablespoons flour

2 cups unsweetened fortified soymilk

2 teaspoons onion powder

1 teaspoon garlic powder

2 tablespoons nutritional yeast

1 teaspoon lemon juice

½ teaspoon salt

¾ teaspoon paprika

½ teaspoon black pepper

¾ cup bread crumbs or French-fried onions (optional)

Folic Acid: 🍎🍎🍎

Vitamin B$_{12}$: 🍎🍎🍎

Protein: 🍎🍎

Iron: 🍎

Zinc: 🍎🍎

Calcium: 🍎🍎

Vitamin D: 🍎

1. Preheat oven to 375°F.
2. Slice potatoes into thin coins and arrange half the slices in a casserole or baking dish. Layer half of the onions on top of the potatoes.
3. Melt the margarine over low heat and add flour, stirring to make a paste. Add soymilk, onion powder, garlic powder, nutritional yeast, lemon juice, and salt, stirring to combine. Stir over low heat until sauce has thickened, about 2–3 minutes.
4. Pour half of sauce over potatoes and onions, then layer the remaining potatoes and onions on top of the sauce. Pour the remaining sauce on top.
5. Sprinkle with paprika and black pepper and top with bread crumbs or French-fried onions.
6. Cover and bake for 45 minutes and then an additional 10 minutes uncovered.

Per Serving
Calories: 264 | Fat: 5g | Sodium: 406mg | Fiber: 7g | Protein: 9g

Green Bean Amandine

Fresh green beans are so much tastier than the frozen or canned variety! Try preparing them with almonds and mushrooms, with this easy, rhyming Green Bean Amandine.

SERVES 4

1 pound fresh green beans, trimmed and chopped

2 tablespoons olive oil

⅓ cup sliced almonds

¾ cup sliced mushrooms

½ yellow onion, chopped

½ teaspoon lemon juice

Folic Acid: 🍎

Vitamin B₁₂: NA

Protein: 🍎

Iron: 🍎

Zinc: 🍎

Calcium: 🍎

Vitamin D: only present in very small amounts

1. Boil green beans in water for just 3–4 minutes; do not overcook. Or steam for 4–5 minutes. Drain and rinse under cold water.
2. In olive oil, sauté almonds, mushrooms, and onion over medium heat for 3–4 minutes, stirring frequently. Add green beans and lemon juice and heat for another minute or two.

Per Serving
Calories: 147 | Fat: 11g | Sodium: 8mg | Fiber: 5g | Protein: 4g

Roasted Brussels Sprouts with Apples

Brussels sprouts are surprisingly delicious when prepared properly, so if you have bad memories of being force-fed soggy, limp baby cabbages as a child, don't let that stop you from trying this recipe!

SERVES 4

2 cups Brussels sprouts, chopped into quarters

8 whole cloves garlic, peeled

2 tablespoons olive oil

2 tablespoons balsamic vinegar

¾ teaspoon salt

½ teaspoon black pepper

2 apples, cored and chopped

Folic Acid: 🍎

Vitamin B$_{12}$: NA

Protein: 🍎

Iron: 🍎

Zinc: 🍎

Calcium: 🍎

Vitamin D: NA

1. Preheat oven to 425°F.
2. Arrange Brussels sprouts and garlic in a single layer on a baking sheet. Drizzle with olive oil and balsamic vinegar and season with salt and pepper. Roast for 10–12 minutes, tossing once.
3. Remove tray from oven and add apples, tossing gently to combine. Roast for 10 more minutes or until apples are soft, tossing once again.

Per Serving
Calories: 143 | Fat: 7g | Sodium: 451mg | Fiber: 4g | Protein: 2g

Reuse and Recycle!

Recycle this basic recipe by adding an extra garnish or two each time you make it: a touch of fresh rosemary, a couple shakes of a vegan Parmesan cheese, some chopped toasted nuts or vegetarian bacon bits for crunch. For a Thanksgiving side dish, toss in some rehydrated dried cranberries.

Saucy Chinese Veggies with Seitan or Tempeh

This is a simple and basic stir-fry recipe with Asian ingredients, suitable for a main dish. Serve over noodles or rice.

SERVES 6

1½ cups vegetable broth

3 tablespoons soy sauce

1 tablespoon rice vinegar

1 teaspoon minced ginger

1 teaspoon sugar

1 (18-ounce) block tempeh, cubed, or about 1 cup chopped seitan

2 tablespoons olive oil

1 red bell pepper, chopped

1 cup snow peas

½ cup sliced water chestnuts (optional)

¼ cup sliced bamboo shoots (optional)

2 scallions, sliced

1 tablespoon cornstarch

Folic Acid: 🍎

Vitamin B₁₂: 🍎

Protein: 🍎🍎🍎

Iron: 🍎

Zinc: 🍎🍎

Calcium: 🍎

Vitamin D: NA

1. In a small bowl, whisk together the vegetable broth, soy sauce, rice vinegar, ginger, and sugar.
2. In a large skillet, brown the tempeh or seitan in olive oil on all sides, about 3–4 minutes.
3. Add bell pepper, snow peas, water chestnuts, bamboo shoots, and scallions, and heat just until vegetables are almost soft, about 2–3 minutes, stirring constantly.
4. Reduce heat and add vegetable broth mixture. Whisk in cornstarch. Bring to a slow simmer and cook until thickened, stirring to prevent lumps.

Per Serving
Calories: 232 | Fat: 14g | Sodium: 700mg | Fiber: 1g | Protein: 16g

Lemon Mint New Potatoes

Potatoes are an easy standby side that goes with just about any entrée, and this version with fresh mint adds a twist to the usual herb-roasted version.

SERVES 4

10–12 small new potatoes, chopped

4 cloves garlic, minced

1 tablespoon olive oil

¼ cup chopped mint

Salt and pepper to taste

2 teaspoons lemon juice

Folic Acid: 🍎🍎

Vitamin B₁₂: NA

Protein: 🍎

Iron: 🍎

Zinc: 🍎

Calcium: 🍎

Vitamin D: NA

1. Preheat oven to 350°F. Line or lightly grease a baking sheet.
2. In a large bowl, toss together the potatoes with the garlic, olive oil, and mint, coating potatoes well.
3. Arrange potatoes in a single layer on a baking sheet. Roast for 45 minutes.
4. Season with salt and pepper and drizzle with lemon juice just before serving.

Per Serving
Calories: 272 | Fat: 4g | Sodium: 23mg | Fiber: 9g | Protein: 6g

Gingered and Pralined Sweet Potatoes

Keep this recipe handy during the holiday season. Who needs marshmallows anyway?

SERVES 4

4 sweet potatoes, baked

¼ cup soy creamer or soymilk

¼ cup orange juice

½ teaspoon salt

½ cup chopped pecans

2 tablespoons vegan margarine

⅓ cup maple syrup

⅓ cup flour

⅓ cup crystallized (candied) ginger

Folic Acid: 🍏

Vitamin B$_{12}$: NA

Protein: 🍏

Iron: 🍏

Zinc: 🍏 🍏

Calcium: 🍏

Vitamin D: NA

① Preheat oven to 350°F.

② Mash together the sweet potatoes, soy creamer or soymilk, orange juice, and salt until smooth and creamy. Transfer to a lightly greased casserole dish.

③ In a small bowl, combine the remaining ingredients and spread over the top of the sweet potatoes.

④ Bake for 30 minutes.

Per Serving
Calories: 436 | Fat: 17g | Sodium: 443mg | Fiber: 6g | Protein: 5g

Why Aren't Marshmallows Vegan?

They aren't even technically vegetarian! Marshmallows contain gelatin, which is extracted from boiled animal bones or hides. Online specialty stores and some natural-foods stores may stock vegan marshmallows, but candied ginger adds an elegant twist to this holiday favorite!

Garlic and Gingered Green Beans

Afraid of vampires? This garlicky recipe ought to scare them away.

SERVES 4

1 pound fresh green beans, trimmed and chopped

2 tablespoons olive oil

4 cloves garlic, minced

1 teaspoon fresh minced ginger

½ teaspoon crushed red pepper flakes

Salt and pepper to taste

Folic Acid: 🍎

Vitamin B$_{12}$: NA

Protein: 🍎

Iron: 🍎

Zinc: 🍎

Calcium: 🍎

Vitamin D: NA

1. Boil green beans in water for just 3–4 minutes; do not overcook. Or steam for 4–5 minutes. Drain and rinse under cold water.
2. Heat olive oil in a skillet with garlic, ginger, green beans, and red pepper flakes. Cook, stirring frequently, for 3–4 minutes until garlic is soft.
3. Taste, and season lightly with salt and pepper.

Per Serving
Calories: 100 | Fat: 7g | Sodium: 8mg | Fiber: 4g | Protein: 2g

Sweetened Roast Squash

Naturally sweet squash is delicious in this simple quick side. Serve as is, scooping it out of the skin, or remove the soft flesh and give it a quick mash.

SERVES 4

1 butternut, acorn, or spaghetti squash

1 teaspoon sea salt

4 tablespoons orange juice

4 tablespoons maple syrup

Nutmeg or ginger to taste

Folic Acid: 🍎

Vitamin B$_{12}$: NA

Protein: 🍎

Iron: 🍎

Zinc: 🍎

Calcium: 🍎

Vitamin D: NA

1. Preheat oven to 400°F.
2. Chop squash into fourths, and scrape out seeds. Place in a large casserole dish. Sprinkle each chunk of squash with a bit of sea salt, 1 teaspoon orange juice, and 1 tablespoon maple syrup, then a shake of nutmeg or ginger.
3. Cover with foil and bake for 40–45 minutes until squash is soft, basting with any extra sauce once or twice.

Per Serving
Calories: 91 | Fat: 0g | Sodium: 586mg | Fiber: 1g | Protein: 1g

Easy Roasted Squash Sides

Tossing squash in the oven couldn't be easier. A drizzle of olive oil and a dash of garlic powder, salt, nutritional yeast, and perhaps a touch of cayenne will also produce a satisfying roasted squash for a side dish you don't need to sweat over.

Classic Green Bean Casserole

Shop for a vegan cream of mushroom soup to use in your traditional holiday recipe, or try this easy homemade vegan version. Delish!

SERVES 4

1 (12-ounce) bag frozen green beans

¾ cup sliced mushrooms

2 tablespoons vegan margarine

2 tablespoons flour

1½ cups plain fortified soymilk

1 tablespoon Dijon mustard

½ teaspoon garlic powder

½ teaspoon salt

¼ teaspoon sage

¼ teaspoon oregano

¼ teaspoon black pepper

1½ cups French-fried onions

Folic Acid: 🍎

Vitamin B$_{12}$: 🍎🍎🍎

Protein: 🍎

Iron: 🍎

Zinc: 🍎

Calcium: 🍎🍎

Vitamin D: 🍎

1. Preheat oven to 375°F. Place green beans and mushrooms in a large casserole dish.
2. Melt vegan margarine over low heat. Stir in flour until pasty and combined. Add soymilk, mustard, garlic powder, salt, sage, oregano, and pepper, stirring continuously to combine until thickened.
3. Pour sauce over mushrooms and green beans and top with French-fried onions.
4. Bake for 16–18 minutes until onions are lightly browned and toasted.

Per Serving
Calories: 279 | Fat: 18g | Sodium: 642mg | Fiber: 3g | Protein: 5g

Caramelized Baby Carrots

Baby carrots have a natural sweetness when cooked, and this recipe turns them into a treat even the pickiest veggie hater will gobble up.

SERVES 4

4 cups baby carrots

1 teaspoon lemon juice

2 tablespoons vegan margarine

2 tablespoons brown sugar

¼ teaspoon sea salt

Folic Acid: 🫑

Vitamin B$_{12}$: NA

Protein: 🫑

Iron: 🫑

Zinc: 🫑

Calcium: 🫑

Vitamin D: NA

1. Simmer carrots in water until just soft, about 8–10 minutes; do not overcook. Drain and drizzle with lemon juice.
2. Heat together carrots, margarine, brown sugar, and sea salt, stirring frequently until glaze forms and carrots are well coated, about 5 minutes.

Per Serving

Calories: 119 | Fat: 6g | Sodium: 322mg | Fiber: 4g | Protein: 1g

Roasted Garlic, Zucchini, and Onions

Roasting veggies brings out their natural flavors, so little additional seasoning is needed in this delicious recipe.

SERVES 4

6 whole cloves garlic

4 zucchini, chopped

1 onion, chopped into rings

1 tablespoon balsamic vinegar

1 tablespoon olive oil

Salt and pepper, to taste

1 teaspoon fresh thyme

2 teaspoons nutritional yeast (optional)

Folic Acid: 🍎🍎

Vitamin B$_{12}$: NA

Protein: 🍎

Iron: 🍎

Zinc: 🍎

Calcium: 🍎

Vitamin D: NA

1. Preheat oven to 400°F.
2. Arrange the garlic, zucchini, and onions on a baking sheet. Drizzle with vinegar and oil and season with salt and pepper, tossing to coat well.
3. Roast in oven for 20–25 minutes, then toss with fresh thyme, nutritional yeast, and additional salt and pepper to taste.

Per Serving
Calories: 83 | Fat: 4g | Sodium: 23mg | Fiber: 3g | Protein: 3g

Cuban Black Beans,
Sweet Potatoes, and Rice

Stir some plain steamed rice right into the pot, or serve it alongside these well-seasoned beans.

SERVES 4

3 cloves garlic, minced

2 large sweet potatoes, peeled and chopped small

2 tablespoons olive oil

2 (15-ounce) cans black beans, drained

¾ cup vegetable broth

1 tablespoon chili powder

1 teaspoon paprika

1 teaspoon cumin

1 tablespoon lime juice

Hot sauce, to taste

2 cups cooked rice

Folic Acid: 🍎🍎🍎

Vitamin B$_{12}$: NA

Protein: 🍎🍎

Iron: 🍎🍎

Zinc: 🍎🍎

Calcium: 🍎

Vitamin D: NA

1. In a large skillet or pot, sauté garlic and sweet potatoes in olive oil for 2–3 minutes.
2. Reduce heat to medium-low and add beans, vegetable broth, chili powder, paprika, and cumin. Bring to a simmer, cover, and allow to cook for 25–30 minutes until sweet potatoes are soft.
3. Stir in lime juice and hot sauce, to taste. Serve hot over rice.

Per Serving
Calories: 387 | Fat: 8g | Sodium: 491mg | Fiber: 13g | Protein: 13g

Spanish Artichoke and Zucchini Paella

Traditional Spanish paellas are always cooked with saffron, but this version with zucchini, artichokes, and bell peppers uses turmeric instead for the same golden hue.

SERVES 4

3 cloves garlic, minced

1 yellow onion, diced

2 tablespoons olive oil

1 cup white rice, uncooked

1 (15-ounce) can diced or crushed tomatoes

1 green bell pepper, chopped

1 red or yellow bell pepper, chopped

½ cup artichoke hearts, chopped

2 zucchini, sliced

2 cups vegetable broth

1 tablespoon paprika

½ teaspoon turmeric

¾ teaspoon parsley

½ teaspoon salt

Folic Acid: 🍎 🍎

Vitamin B$_{12}$: NA

Protein: 🍎

Iron: 🍎 🍎

Zinc: 🍎

Calcium: 🍎

Vitamin D: NA

1. In the largest skillet you can find, heat garlic and onions in olive oil for 3–4 minutes until onions are almost soft. Add rice, stirring well to coat, and heat for another minute, stirring to prevent burning.
2. Add tomatoes, bell peppers, artichokes, and zucchini, stirring to combine. Add vegetable broth and remaining ingredients, cover, and simmer for 15–20 minutes, or until rice is done.

Per Serving
Calories: 260 | Fat: 1g | Sodium: 1,016mg | Fiber: 6g | Protein: 7g

Chinese Fried Rice with Tofu and Cashews

On busy weeknights, pick up some plain white rice from a Chinese take-out restaurant and turn it into a home-cooked meal in a jiffy. Garnish with fresh lime wedges and a sprinkle of sea salt and fresh black pepper on top.

SERVES 4

2 cloves garlic, minced

1 (12-ounce) block silken tofu, mashed with a fork

3 tablespoons olive oil

3 cups leftover cooked rice

½ cup frozen mixed diced veggies

3 tablespoons soy sauce

1 tablespoon sesame oil

2 tablespoons lime juice

3 scallions (greens and whites), sliced

⅓ cup chopped cashews (optional)

Folic Acid: 🍎🍎

Vitamin B$_{12}$: NA

Protein: 🍎🍎

Iron: 🍎🍎

Zinc: 🍎🍎

Calcium: 🍎

Vitamin D: NA

① In a large skillet or wok, sauté the garlic and tofu in 2 tablespoons olive oil over medium-high heat, stirring frequently, until tofu is lightly browned, about 6–8 minutes.

② Add remaining 1 tablespoon olive oil, rice, and veggies, stirring well to combine.

③ Add soy sauce and sesame oil and combine well.

④ Allow to cook, stirring constantly, for 3–4 minutes.

⑤ Remove from heat and stir in remaining ingredients.

Per Serving
Calories: 358 | Fat: 16g | Sodium: 723mg | Fiber: 2g | Protein: 11g

Quick Healthy Meals

Like stir-fries and an easy pasta recipe, fried rice is a quick and easy meal you can turn to again and again. The formula is always the same: rice, oil, and seasonings, but the variations are endless. Besides tofu, try adding tempeh, seitan, or store-bought mock meats to fried rice. Add kimchi for a Korean spice, or season with a mixture of cumin, curry, ginger, and turmeric for an Indian-inspired dish.

Mushroom and Rosemary Wild Rice

Top this recipe off with some Lemon Basil Tofu slices (see recipe in Chapter 5) for an herb-infused main dish.

SERVES 4

1 tablespoon chopped fresh rosemary

1 yellow onion, diced

2 tablespoons olive oil

1 cup sliced mushrooms

1½ cups wild rice, uncooked

4½ cups vegetable broth

2 tablespoons vegan margarine

½ teaspoon lemon juice

¼ teaspoon ground sage

2 tablespoons nutritional yeast

Folic Acid: 🍎🍎🍎

Vitamin B$_{12}$: 🍎🍎🍎

Protein: 🍎🍎

Iron: 🍎

Zinc: 🍎🍎🍎

Calcium: 🍎

Vitamin D: only present in very small amounts

1. In a large pan, heat rosemary and onion in olive oil until onions are just soft, about 3 minutes. Add mushrooms, and heat for another minute.
2. Add wild rice and vegetable broth and bring to a simmer. Cover and cook 40–45 minutes until rice is done and liquid is absorbed.
3. Remove from heat and stir in remaining ingredients.

Per Serving
Calories: 366 | Fat: 13g | Sodium: 1,145mg | Fiber: 5g | Protein: 11g

Indian Lemon Rice Pilaf

With an unexpected blend of flavors, lemon rice is a popular favorite to serve to the gods and their devotees in South Indian temples. Kick up the heat by adding a couple green chilies, or, if you can find them at an Indian grocer, heat some dried curry leaves with the mustard seeds.

SERVES 4

1½ teaspoons black mustard seeds

2 tablespoons olive oil

½ teaspoon turmeric

1 cup rice, uncooked

1¾ cups vegetable broth or water

½ cup frozen peas

2 tablespoons lemon juice

¼ cup yellow raisins

2 tablespoons scallions, chopped

2 tablespoons chopped fresh cilantro (optional)

Folic Acid: 🍎🍎

Vitamin B$_{12}$: NA

Protein: 🍎

Iron: 🍎

Zinc: 🍎

Calcium: 🍎

Vitamin D: NA

1. Heat mustard seeds in olive oil over medium heat for about 1 minute.
2. Add turmeric and rice and stir well to combine. Toast rice, stirring, for 1–2 minutes until lightly golden brown.
3. Add vegetable broth or water and bring to a slow simmer. Cover and allow to cook for about 15 minutes until rice is done.
4. Reduce heat to medium-low and add peas and lemon juice, cooking for another minute or two until peas are heated through.
5. Remove from heat and stir in remaining ingredients.

Per Serving
Calories: 283 | Fat: 8g | Sodium: 434mg | Fiber: 2g | Protein: 5g

Squash and Sage Risotto

Risotto is easy to make, but it does take a bit of effort with all the stirring! This earthy recipe works well with just about any kind of squash. If you're in a hurry, use canned puréed pumpkin instead of fresh acorn squash or look for precooked butternut squash in your grocer's freezer section.

SERVES 4

3 cloves garlic, minced

½ yellow onion, diced

2 tablespoons olive oil

1½ cups Arborio rice, uncooked

5 cups vegetable broth

2 whole cloves

1½ cups roasted puréed pumpkin, acorn, or butternut squash

1½ teaspoons sage

⅓ teaspoon salt

¼ teaspoon pepper

Folic Acid: 🍎🍎🍎

Vitamin B$_{12}$: NA

Protein: 🍎

Iron: 🍎🍎🍎

Zinc: 🍎

Calcium: 🍎

Vitamin D: NA

① In a large skillet, sauté the garlic and onions in olive oil for 3 minutes over medium-high heat. Add uncooked rice and cook for 2 more minutes, stirring frequently to lightly toast the rice.

② Add ¾ cup vegetable broth and cloves and stir well. When most of the liquid has been absorbed, add another ½ cup broth, stirring frequently. Continue adding vegetable broth ½ cup at a time until rice is just tender and sauce is creamy, about 20–25 minutes. Reduce heat to medium-low and stir in puréed squash and ¼ cup vegetable broth. Continue to stir well and allow to cook for 4–5 more minutes.

③ Stir in sage and season with salt and pepper.

④ Allow to cool, stirring occasionally, for at least 5 minutes. Risotto will thicken slightly as it cools. Remove cloves before serving.

Per Serving
Calories: 371 | Fat: 7g | Sodium: 1,370mg | Fiber: 4g | Protein: 6g

Indonesian Fried Rice (Nasi Goreng)

You might like some diced veggie dogs in this recipe, instead of or alongside the tempeh. Like any fried rice recipe, the vegetables you use are really up to you.

SERVES 6

2 teaspoons molasses

2 tablespoons soy sauce

1 (18-ounce) block tempeh, cubed

1 onion, diced

3 cloves garlic, minced

1 small chili, minced

3–4 tablespoons vegetable oil or peanut oil

3 cups cooked rice

1 tablespoon sesame oil

2 tablespoons ketchup

2 tablespoons hot chili sauce

2 scallions, chopped

1 carrot, sliced thin

1 red or yellow bell pepper, diced

Dash Chinese five-spice powder (optional)

Folic Acid: 🍎

Vitamin B$_{12}$: NA

Protein: 🍎🍎

Iron: 🍎

Zinc: 🍎

Calcium: 🍎

Vitamin D: NA

1. Whisk together the molasses and soy sauce, and set aside.
2. In a large skillet, sauté the tempeh, onion, garlic, and chili in oil for a few minutes until tempeh is lightly browned. Add rice and sesame oil, stirring to combine.
3. Add remaining ingredients, including molasses and soy sauce, and quickly stir to combine.
4. Cook for just a few minutes, stirring constantly, until heated through.

Per Serving
Calories: 296 | Fat: 13g | Sodium: 433mg | Fiber: 2g | Protein: 10g

Caribbean Red Beans and Rice

Cook the beans from scratch and use the cooking liquid instead of the vegetable broth if you've got the time.

SERVES 6

3 cloves garlic, peeled

1 small onion, chopped

3 ribs celery, chopped

2 tablespoons chopped fresh parsley

2 tablespoons olive oil

½ teaspoon rosemary

½ teaspoon thyme

¼ teaspoon cloves

1 (15-ounce) can kidney beans, drained

3 cups vegetable broth

2 bay leaves

1½ cups rice, uncooked

Dash salt and pepper to taste

Folic Acid: 🍎🍎🍎

Vitamin B$_{12}$: NA

Protein: 🍎

Iron: 🍎🍎

Zinc: 🍎

Calcium: 🍎

Vitamin D: NA

① Use a food processor to process the garlic, onion, celery, and parsley until finely grated or minced.

② Heat onion mixture in olive oil in a skillet, stirring frequently, for a few minutes until soft. Add rosemary, thyme, cloves, and beans, stirring to combine well. Cook for a few more minutes until fragrant.

③ Reduce heat and add vegetable broth, bay leaves, and rice. Bring to a slow simmer, cover, and cook for 30 minutes.

④ Reduce heat to low, uncover, and cook for 10 more minutes, or until most of the liquid is absorbed. Season with salt and pepper.

⑤ Remove bay leaves before serving.

Per Serving
Calories: 430 | Fat: 8g | Sodium: 1,046mg | Fiber: 8g | Protein: 11g

Cranberry Apple Wild Rice

To speed up the cooking time, soak the wild rice for 15–20 minutes before boiling.

SERVES 4

1 rib celery, diced

1 red onion, diced

2 tablespoons olive oil

1 cup wild rice

3 cups water or vegetable broth

⅓ cup orange juice

½ cup dried cranberries or raisins

½ cup pine nuts or sliced almonds

2 scallions, chopped

1 apple, diced

Salt and pepper to taste

Folic Acid: 🍎🍎

Vitamin B$_{12}$: NA

Protein: 🍎🍎

Iron: 🍎

Zinc: 🍎🍎🍎

Calcium: 🍎

Vitamin D: NA

1. In a large soup or stockpot, sauté celery and onion in olive oil for 3–4 minutes until soft.
2. Reduce heat and add wild rice and water or vegetable broth. Bring to a simmer, cover, and cook for 30 minutes. Add orange juice, and simmer for another 10–15 minutes, or until rice is cooked.
3. Remove from heat and add cranberries. Cover and let sit for 5 minutes.
4. Toss with remaining ingredients and serve hot or cold.

Per Serving
Calories: 427 | Fat: 19g | Sodium: 721mg | Fiber: 6g | Protein: 10g

Baked Mexican Rice Casserole

This is a quick and easy side dish you can get into the oven in just a few minutes.

SERVES 4

1 (15-ounce) can black beans

¾ cup salsa

2 teaspoons chili powder

1 teaspoon cumin

½ cup corn kernels

2 cups cooked rice

½ cup grated vegan cheese (optional)

⅓ cup sliced black olives

Folic Acid: 🍎🍎🍎

Vitamin B₁₂: NA

Protein: 🍎🍎

Iron: 🍎🍎

Zinc: 🍎🍎

Calcium: 🍎

Vitamin D: NA

1. Preheat oven to 350°F.
2. Combine the beans, salsa, chili powder, and cumin in a large pot over low heat, and partially mash beans with a large fork.
3. Remove from heat and stir in corn and rice. Transfer to a casserole dish.
4. Top with vegan cheese and sliced olives and bake for 20 minutes.

Per Serving
Calories: 289 | Fat: 2g | Sodium: 539mg | Fiber: 11g | Protein: 13g

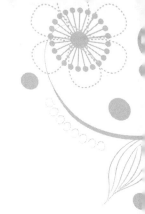

CHAPTER 7

Salads
and Vegetables

Carrot and Date Salad

If you're used to carrot and raisin salads drowning in mayonnaise, this lighter version with tahini, dates, and mandarin oranges will be a welcome change.

SERVES 4

⅓ cup tahini

1 tablespoon olive oil

2 tablespoons agave nectar or 2 teaspoons sugar

3 tablespoons lemon juice

¼ teaspoon salt

4 large carrots, grated

½ cup chopped dates

3 Satsuma or mandarin oranges, sectioned

⅓ cup coconut flakes (optional)

Folic Acid: 🍎

Vitamin B₁₂: NA

Protein: 🍎

Iron: 🍎

Zinc: 🍎

Calcium: 🍎🍎

Vitamin D: NA

① In a small bowl, whisk together the tahini, olive oil, agave nectar, lemon juice, and salt.

② Place grated carrots in a large bowl; toss well with tahini mixture.

③ Add dates, oranges, and coconut flakes; combine well.

④ Allow to sit for at least 1 hour before serving to soften carrots and dates. Toss again before serving.

Per Serving
Calories: 307 | Fat: 15g | Sodium: 220mg | Fiber: 7g | Protein: 5g

Edamame Salad

If you can't find shelled edamame, try this recipe with lima beans instead.

SERVES 4

2 cups frozen shelled edamame, thawed and drained

1 red or yellow bell pepper, diced

¾ cup corn kernels, fresh or frozen and thawed

3 tablespoons chopped fresh cilantro (optional)

3 tablespoons olive oil

2 tablespoons red wine vinegar

1 teaspoon soy sauce

1 teaspoon chili powder

2 teaspoons lemon or lime juice

Salt and pepper, to taste

Folic Acid: 🍎
Vitamin B$_{12}$: NA
Protein: 🍎🍎
Iron: 🍎
Zinc: 🍎
Calcium: 🍎
Vitamin D: NA

1. In a large bowl, combine edamame, bell pepper, corn, and cilantro.
2. Whisk together the olive oil, vinegar, soy sauce, chili powder, and lemon juice; combine with the edamame. Add salt and pepper, to taste.
3. Chill for at least 1 hour before serving.

Per Serving
Calories: 246 | Fat: 16g | Sodium: 133mg | Fiber: 9g | Protein: 10g

Italian White Bean and Fresh Herb Salad

Don't let the simplicity of this bean salad fool you! The fresh herbs marinate the beans to flavorful perfection, so there's no need to add anything else!

SERVES 4

2 (15-ounce) cans cannellini or great Northern beans, drained and rinsed

2 ribs celery, diced

¼ cup chopped fresh parsley

¼ cup chopped fresh basil

3 tablespoons olive oil

3 large tomatoes, chopped

½ cup sliced black olives

2 tablespoons lemon juice

Salt and pepper, to taste

¼ teaspoon crushed red pepper flakes (optional)

Folic Acid: 🍎🍎🍎

Vitamin B$_{12}$: NA

Protein: 🍎🍎🍎

Iron: 🍎🍎🍎

Zinc: 🍎🍎🍎

Calcium: 🍎🍎

Vitamin D: NA

1. In a large skillet, combine the beans, celery, parsley, and basil with olive oil. Heat, stirring frequently, over low heat for 3 minutes, until herbs are softened but not cooked.
2. Remove from heat; stir in remaining ingredients, gently tossing to combine. Chill for at least 1 hour before serving.

Per Serving
Calories: 377 | Fat: 14g | Sodium: 279mg | Fiber: 12g | Protein: 16g

Kidney Bean and Chickpea Salad

This marinated two-bean salad is perfect for summer picnics or as a side for outdoor barbecues or baby showers.

SERVES 6

¼ cup olive oil

¼ cup red wine vinegar

½ teaspoon paprika

2 tablespoons lemon juice

1 (15-ounce) can chickpeas, drained and rinsed

1 (15-ounce) can kidney beans, drained and rinsed

½ cup sliced black olives

1 (8-ounce) can corn, drained

½ red onion, chopped

1 tablespoon chopped fresh parsley

Salt and pepper, to taste

Folic Acid: 🍎🍎

Vitamin B$_{12}$: NA

Protein: 🍎

Iron: 🍎

Zinc: 🍎🍎

Calcium: 🍎

Vitamin D: NA

1. Whisk together olive oil, vinegar, paprika, and lemon juice.
2. In a large bowl, combine the chickpeas, beans, olives, corn, onion, and parsley. Pour the dressing over the bean mixture; toss well to combine.
3. Season generously with salt and pepper, to taste.
4. Chill for at least 1 hour before serving to allow flavors to mingle.

Per Serving
Calories: 252 | Fat: 12g | Sodium: 569mg | Fiber: 8g | Protein: 7g

Lemon-Cumin Potato Salad

A mayonnaise-free potato salad with exotic flavors, this one is delicious either hot or cold.

SERVES 4

2 tablespoons olive oil

1 small yellow onion, diced

1½ teaspoons cumin

4 large cooked potatoes, chopped

3 tablespoons lemon juice

2 teaspoons Dijon mustard

1 scallion, chopped

¼ teaspoon cayenne pepper

2 tablespoons chopped fresh cilantro (optional)

Folic Acid: 🍎🍎

Vitamin B$_{12}$: NA

Protein: 🍎🍎

Iron: 🍎🍎

Zinc: 🍎🍎

Calcium: 🍎

Vitamin D: NA

① In a skillet over medium heat, add the olive oil. Once the oil is warm, add onions and cook until soft, about 5 minutes.

② Add cumin and potatoes; cook for just 1 minute, stirring well to combine. Remove from heat.

③ Whisk together the lemon juice and Dijon mustard; pour over potatoes, tossing gently to coat.

④ Add scallions, cayenne pepper, and cilantro; combine well.

⑤ Chill before serving.

Per Serving
Calories: 360 | Fat: 7g | Sodium: 53mg | Fiber: 9g | Protein: 8g

No-Mayo Apple Coleslaw

There's nothing wrong with grabbing a store-bought, preshredded coleslaw mix from the produce section to make this vegan salad, just double the dressing if you find it's not enough.

SERVES 4

1 head cabbage, shredded

1 apple, diced small

1 (15-ounce) can pineapple, drained, 2 tablespoons juice reserved

1 tablespoon apple cider vinegar

2 tablespoons olive oil

1 tablespoon tahini

2 tablespoons agave nectar or 1 teaspoon sugar

2 tablespoons sunflower seeds (optional)

Folic Acid: 🍎🍎

Vitamin B$_{12}$: NA

Protein: 🍎

Iron: 🍎

Zinc: 🍎

Calcium: 🍎🍎

Vitamin D: NA

1. In a large bowl, combine the cabbage, apple, and pineapple.
2. In a separate small bowl, whisk together 2 tablespoons of the pineapple juice with the cider vinegar, olive oil, and tahini. Pour over cabbage and apples; toss gently to coat.
3. Drizzle with agave nectar; toss to coat.
4. Chill for at least 30 minutes before serving. Toss with sunflower seeds.

Per Serving
Calories: 196 | Fat: 2g | Sodium: 47mg | Fiber: 8g | Protein: 4g

Spicy Sweet Cucumber Salad

Japanese cucumber salad is cool and refreshing, but with a bit of spice. Enjoy it as a healthy afternoon snack or as a fresh accompaniment to take-out.

SERVES 2

2 cucumbers, sliced thin

¾ teaspoon salt

¼ cup rice wine vinegar

1 teaspoon sugar or 1 tablespoon agave nectar

1 teaspoon sesame oil

¼ teaspoon red pepper flakes

½ onion, sliced thin

Folic Acid: 🍎

Vitamin B₁₂: NA

Protein: 🍎

Iron: 🍎

Zinc: 🍎

Calcium: 🍎

Vitamin D: NA

1. In a large shallow container or baking sheet, spread the cucumbers in a single layer; sprinkle with salt. Allow to sit at least 10 minutes.
2. Drain any excess water from the cucumbers.
3. Whisk together the rice wine vinegar, sugar, oil, and red pepper flakes.
4. Pour dressing over the cucumbers; add onions, and toss gently.
5. Allow to sit at least 10 minutes before serving to allow flavors to mingle.

Per Serving
Calories: 90 | Fat: 3g | Sodium: 880mg | Fiber: 2g | Protein: 2g

Dairy-Free Ranch Dressing

This recipe is for an all-American creamy homemade ranch dressing, without the buttermilk. Get those baby carrots ready to dip!

YIELDS 1 CUP

1 (12-ounce) block silken tofu

2½ tablespoons lemon juice

1 teaspoon prepared yellow mustard

1½ teaspoons apple cider or white vinegar

1 teaspoon sugar

½ teaspoon salt

⅓ cup canola or safflower oil

¼ cup fortified soymilk

1 teaspoon Dijon mustard

1¾ teaspoons onion powder

¾ teaspoon garlic powder

1 tablespoon minced fresh chives

Folic Acid: only present in very small amounts

Vitamin B$_{12}$: NA

Protein: 🍎

Iron: NA

Zinc: NA

Calcium: only present in very small amounts

Vitamin D: only present in very small amounts

① In a food processor, process tofu, lemon juice, mustard, vinegar, sugar, and salt until smooth.

② On high speed, slowly incorporate the oil just a few drops at a time, until smooth and creamy.

③ Whisk or blend in remaining ingredients except chives until smooth, then stir in chives until well combined.

Per Tablespoon
Calories: 57 | Fat: 5g | Sodium: 83mg | Fiber: 0g | Protein: 1g

Thai Orange Peanut Dressing

This recipe is a sweet and spicy take on traditional Thai and Indonesian peanut and satay sauce. Add a bit less liquid to use this salad dressing as a dip for veggies.

YIELDS ¾ CUP

¼ cup peanut butter, at room temperature

¼ cup orange juice

2 tablespoons soy sauce

2 tablespoons rice vinegar

2 tablespoons water

½ teaspoon garlic powder

½ teaspoon sugar

¼ teaspoon crushed red pepper flakes (optional)

Folic Acid: 🌶

Vitamin B$_{12}$: NA

Protein: 🌶

Iron: only present in very small amounts

Zinc: 🌶

Calcium: only present in very small amounts

Vitamin D: NA

● Whisk together all ingredients until smooth and creamy, adding more or less liquid to achieve desired consistency.

Per Tablespoon
Calories: 36 | Fat: 3g | Sodium: 176mg | Fiber: 0g | Protein: 1g

Goddess Dressing

Turn this zesty salad dressing into a dip for veggies or a sandwich spread by reducing the amount of liquids.

YIELDS 1½ CUPS

⅔ cup tahini

¼ cup apple cider vinegar

⅓ cup soy sauce

2 teaspoons lemon juice

1 clove garlic

¾ teaspoon sugar (optional)

⅓ cup olive oil

Folic Acid: only present in very small amounts

Vitamin B$_{12}$: NA

Protein: 🍎

Iron: 🍎

Zinc: 🍎

Calcium: 🍎

Vitamin D: NA

1. In a blender or food processor, process all the ingredients except olive oil until blended.
2. With the blender or food processor on high speed, slowly add in the olive oil, blending for a full minute to allow the oil to emulsify.
3. Chill in the refrigerator for at least 10 minutes before serving; dressing will thicken as it chills.

Per Tablespoon
Calories: 70 | Fat: 7g | Sodium: 208mg | Fiber: 1g | Protein: 1g

In Search of Tahini

Tahini is a sesame seed paste native to Middle Eastern cuisine with a thinner consistency and milder flavor than peanut butter. You'll find a jarred or canned version in the ethnic foods aisle of large grocery stores.

Baked Sweet Potato Fries

Brown sugar adds a sweet touch to these yummy sweet potato fries. If you like your fries with a kick, add some crushed red pepper flakes or a dash of cayenne pepper to the mix.

SERVES 3

2 large sweet potatoes, peeled and sliced into fries

2 tablespoons olive oil

¼ teaspoon garlic powder

½ teaspoon paprika

½ teaspoon brown sugar

½ teaspoon chili powder

¼ teaspoon salt

Folic Acid: 🍎

Vitamin B$_{12}$: NA

Protein: 🍎

Iron: 🍎

Zinc: 🍎

Calcium: 🍎

Vitamin D: NA

1. Preheat oven to 400°F.
2. Spread sweet potatoes on a large baking sheet; drizzle with olive oil, tossing gently to coat.
3. In a small bowl, combine remaining ingredients. Sprinkle over potatoes; coat evenly and toss as needed.
4. Bake in oven for 10 minutes, turning once. Taste, and add more salt, to taste.

Per Serving
Calories: 203 | Fat: 9g | Sodium: 270mg | Fiber: 4g | Protein: 2g

Cajun Collard Greens

Collard greens are a great choice to add calcium and iron to your diet. Add some zesty Cajun seasonings to make them even more appealing.

SERVES 4

1 onion, diced

3 cloves garlic, minced

1 pound collard greens, chopped

2 tablespoons olive oil

¾ cup water or vegetable broth

1 (14-ounce) can diced tomatoes, drained

1½ teaspoons Cajun seasoning

½ teaspoon hot sauce, or to taste

¼ teaspoon salt, or to taste

Folic Acid: 🍎🍎🍎

Vitamin B₁₂: NA

Protein: 🍎

Iron: 🍎

Zinc: 🍎

Calcium: 🍎🍎

Vitamin D: NA

1. In a large skillet, sauté onions, garlic, and collard greens in olive oil for 3–5 minutes, until onions are soft.
2. Add water, tomatoes, and Cajun seasoning. Bring to a simmer; cover, and allow to cook for 20 minutes, or until greens are soft, stirring occasionally.
3. Remove lid, and stir in hot sauce and salt; cook, uncovered, for 1–2 minutes, to allow excess moisture to evaporate.

Per Serving
Calories: 125 | Fat: 7g | Sodium: 517mg | Fiber: 6g | Protein: 4g

Creamed Spinach and Mushrooms

The combination of greens and nutritional yeast is simply delicious and provides an excellent jolt of nutrients that vegans need. Don't forget that spinach will shrink when cooked, so use lots!

SERVES 4

½ onion, diced

2 cloves garlic, minced

1½ cups sliced mushrooms

2 tablespoons olive oil

1 tablespoon flour

2 bunches fresh spinach, trimmed

1 cup plain or unsweetened fortified soymilk

1 tablespoon vegan margarine

¼ teaspoon nutmeg (optional)

2 tablespoons nutritional yeast (optional)

Salt and pepper, to taste

Folic Acid: 🍎🍎🍎

Vitamin B$_{12}$: 🍎🍎🍎

Protein: 🍎

Iron: 🍎🍎

Zinc: 🍎🍎

Calcium: 🍎🍎🍎

Vitamin D: 🍎

1. Sauté onion, garlic, and mushrooms in olive oil for 3–4 minutes. Add flour; heat, stirring constantly, for 1 minute.
2. Reduce heat to medium low; add spinach and soymilk. Cook uncovered for 8–10 minutes, until spinach is soft and liquid has reduced.
3. Stir in remaining ingredients; season with salt and pepper, to taste.

Per Serving
Calories: 169 | Fat: 11g | Sodium: 206mg | Fiber: 5g | Protein: 8g

Summer Squash Sauté

Green zucchini and yellow squash absorb flavors like magic, though little enhancement is needed with their fresh natural flavor. Toss these veggies with some cooked orzo or linguini to make it a main dish.

SERVES 2

1 onion, chopped

2 cloves garlic, minced

2 tablespoons olive oil

2 zucchini, sliced into coins

2 yellow squash, sliced thin

1 large tomato, diced

2 teaspoons Italian seasoning

1 tablespoon nutritional yeast

2 teaspoons hot chili sauce (optional)

Folic Acid: 🍎🍎🍎

Vitamin B$_{12}$: 🍎🍎🍎

Protein: 🍎

Iron: 🍎

Zinc: 🍎🍎

Calcium: 🍎

Vitamin D: NA

1. In a large skillet over medium heat, sauté onions and garlic in olive oil for 1–2 minutes.
2. Add zucchini, squash, and tomato. Heat, stirring frequently, for 4–5 minutes, until squash is soft.
3. Season with Italian seasoning; heat for 1 minute. Stir in yeast and hot sauce.

Per Serving
Calories: 205 | Fat: 14g | Sodium: 28mg | Fiber: 5g | Protein: 5g

Gingered Bok Choy and Tofu Stir-Fry

Dark, leafy bok choy is a highly nutritious vegetable that can be found in well-stocked groceries. Keep an eye out for light-green baby bok choy, which is a bit more tender but carries a similar flavor.

SERVES 4

3 tablespoons soy sauce

2 tablespoons lemon or lime juice

1 tablespoon minced fresh ginger

1 (16-ounce) block firm or extra-firm tofu, well pressed

2 tablespoons olive oil

1 head bok choy or 3–4 small baby bok choy, chopped

½ teaspoon sugar

½ teaspoon sesame oil

Folic Acid: 🍎🍎🍎

Vitamin B₁₂: NA

Protein: 🍎🍎

Iron: 🍎🍎

Zinc: 🍎

Calcium: 🍎🍎🍎

Vitamin D: NA

1. In a shallow pan, whisk together soy sauce, lemon juice, and ginger.
2. Cut tofu into cubes; marinate in the refrigerator for at least 1 hour. Drain, reserving marinade.
3. In a large skillet or wok, sauté tofu in olive oil for 3–4 minutes.
4. Carefully add reserved marinade, bok choy, and sugar; stir well to combine.
5. Cook, stirring, for 3–4 more minutes.
6. Drizzle with sesame oil. Serve over rice.

Per Serving
Calories: 213 | Fat: 15g | Sodium: 1,097mg | Fiber: 4g | Protein: 14g

Maple-Glazed Roasted Veggies

These easy roasted veggies make an excellent holiday side dish. The vegetables can be roasted in advance and reheated with the glaze to save on time, if needed. If parsnips are too earthy for you, substitute one large potato.

SERVES 4

3 carrots, peeled and chopped

2 small parsnips, peeled and chopped

2 sweet potatoes, peeled and chopped

2 tablespoons olive oil

Salt and pepper, to taste

⅓ cup maple syrup

2 tablespoons Dijon mustard

1 tablespoon balsamic vinegar

½ teaspoon hot sauce

Folic Acid: 🍎

Vitamin B₁₂: NA

Protein: 🍎

Iron: 🍎

Zinc: 🍎🍎

Calcium: 🍎

Vitamin D: NA

1. Preheat oven to 400°F.
2. On a large baking sheet, spread out carrots, parsnips, and sweet potatoes.
3. Drizzle with olive oil and season to taste with salt and pepper. Roast for 40 minutes, tossing once.
4. In a small bowl, whisk together syrup, mustard, vinegar, and hot sauce.
5. Transfer the roasted vegetables to a large bowl; toss well with the maple mixture. Add salt and pepper, to taste.

Per Serving
Calories: 231 | Fat: 7g | Sodium: 158mg | Fiber: 5g | Protein: 5g

Orange and Ginger Mixed-Veggie Stir-Fry

Rice vinegar can be substituted for the apple cider vinegar, if you prefer. As with most stir-fry recipes, the vegetables are merely a suggestion; use your favorites or whatever looks like it's been sitting too long in your crisper.

SERVES 4

3 tablespoons orange juice

1 tablespoon apple cider vinegar

2 tablespoons soy sauce

2 tablespoons water

1 tablespoon maple syrup

1 teaspoon powdered ginger

2 tablespoons oil

2 cloves garlic, minced

1 bunch broccoli, chopped

½ cup sliced mushrooms

½ cup snap peas, chopped

1 carrot, sliced

1 cup chopped cabbage or bok choy

Folic Acid:

Vitamin B$_{12}$: NA

Protein:

Iron:

Zinc:

Calcium:

Vitamin D: only present in very small amounts

① Whisk together the orange juice, vinegar, soy sauce, water, maple syrup, and ginger.

② Heat oil in a large skillet, add garlic and cook for 1–2 minutes; add veggies. Allow to cook over high heat, stirring frequently, for 2–3 minutes, until just starting to get tender.

③ Add sauce and reduce heat; simmer, stirring frequently, for another 3–4 minutes, or until veggies are cooked.

Per Serving
Calories: 117 | Fat: 3g | Sodium: 518mg | Fiber: 6g | Protein: 6g

Roasted-Garlic Mashed Potatoes

In the absence of milk and butter, load your mashed potatoes up with roasted garlic for a flavor blast.

SERVES 4

1 whole head garlic

2 tablespoons olive oil

6 potatoes, cooked

¼ cup vegan margarine

½ cup soy creamer or soymilk

Salt and pepper, to taste

Folic Acid: 🍎

Vitamin B$_{12}$: NA

Protein: 🍎

Iron: 🍎

Zinc: 🍎

Calcium: 🍎

Vitamin D: NA

1. Heat oven to 400°F.
2. Remove outer layer of skin from garlic head. Drizzle generously with olive oil, wrap in aluminum foil, and place on a baking sheet. Roast in oven for 30 minutes.
3. Gently press cloves out of the skins; mash smooth with a fork.
4. Using a mixer or a potato masher, combine garlic with potatoes, margarine, and creamer until smooth.
5. Season to taste with salt and pepper.

Per Serving
Calories: 367 | Fat: 14g | Sodium: 199mg | Fiber: 8g | Protein: 6g

Sweet Pineapple Cabbage Stir-Fry

Toss in a can of pineapple the last minute or two to just about any stir-fry recipe for a sweet treat.

SERVES 6

1 (15-ounce) can diced pineapple

2 tablespoons red wine vinegar

1 tablespoon soy sauce

1 tablespoon brown sugar

2 teaspoons cornstarch

¼ teaspoon crushed red pepper flakes

2 tablespoons olive oil

2 cloves garlic, minced

1 onion, chopped

1 head broccoli, chopped

1 head Napa cabbage or ½ head green cabbage, chopped

1 batch Easy Fried Tofu (optional) (see Chapter 5)

Folic Acid: 🍎🍎

Vitamin B$_{12}$: NA

Protein: 🍎

Iron: 🍎

Zinc: 🍎

Calcium: 🍎🍎

Vitamin D: NA

① Drain pineapple, reserving juice. In a medium bowl, whisk together pineapple juice, vinegar, soy sauce, brown sugar, cornstarch, and red pepper flakes.

② In a large skillet heat olive oil, add garlic and onion and cook just until soft, about 3–4 minutes.

③ Add broccoli, pineapple, and cabbage. Stir quickly to combine; cook for 1 minute.

④ Reduce heat to medium; add pineapple juice mixture. Bring to a slow simmer; heat just until mixture has thickened, about 3–5 minutes, stirring frequently.

⑤ Stir in fried tofu. Serve over rice or whole grains.

Per Serving
Calories: 132 | Fat: 5g | Sodium: 252mg | Fiber: 3g | Protein: 4g

Mango and Bell Pepper Stir-Fry

Add some marinated tofu to make it a main dish, or enjoy just the mango and veggies for a light lunch. Thaw frozen cubed mango if you can't find fresh.

SERVES 4

2 tablespoons lime juice

2 tablespoons orange juice

1 tablespoon hot chili sauce

3 tablespoons soy sauce

2 cloves garlic, minced

2 tablespoons oil

1 red bell pepper

1 yellow or orange bell pepper

1 bunch broccoli, chopped

1 mango, cubed

3 scallions, chopped

Folic Acid: 🍎🍎🍎

Vitamin B$_{12}$: NA

Protein: 🍎

Iron: 🍎

Zinc: 🍎

Calcium: 🍎

Vitamin D: NA

1. Whisk together the lime juice, orange juice, hot sauce, and soy sauce.
2. Heat garlic in oil for just a minute or two then add bell peppers and broccoli and cook, stirring frequently, for another 2–3 minutes.
3. Add juice and soy sauce mixture, reduce heat, and cook for another 2–3 minutes until broccoli and bell peppers are almost soft.
4. Reduce heat to low, and add mango and scallions, gently stirring to combine. Heat for just another minute or two until mango is warmed.

Per Serving
Calories: 189 | Fat: 8g | Sodium: 733mg | Fiber: 7g | Protein: 7g

Fiery Basil and Eggplant Stir-Fry

Holy basil, called tulsi, is revered in Vishnu temples across India and is frequently used in Ayurvedic healing. It lends a fantastically spicy flavor, but regular basil will also do.

SERVES 3

3 cloves garlic, minced

3 small fresh chili peppers, minced

1 (16-ounce) block firm or extra-firm tofu, pressed and diced

2 tablespoons olive oil

1 eggplant, chopped

1 red bell pepper, chopped

⅓ cup sliced mushrooms

3 tablespoons water

2 tablespoons soy sauce

1 teaspoon lemon juice

⅓ cup fresh Thai basil or holy basil

Folic Acid: 🍎🍎

Vitamin B₁₂: NA

Protein: 🍎🍎

Iron: 🍎🍎

Zinc: 🍎🍎

Calcium: 🍎

Vitamin D: only present in very small amounts

1. Sauté the garlic, chili peppers, and tofu in olive oil for 4–6 minutes until tofu is lightly golden.
2. Add eggplant, bell pepper, mushrooms, water, and soy sauce and heat, stirring frequently, for 5–6 minutes, or until eggplant is almost soft.
3. Add lemon juice and basil and cook for another minute or two, just until basil is wilted.

Per Serving
Calories: 241 | Fat: 14g | Sodium: 624mg | Fiber: 9g | Protein: 13g

CHAPTER 8

Soups and Stews

"Chicken" Noodle Soup

If you think you're getting a cold—or if you just need something to make you feel better—this vegan soup is even more comforting and delicious than its nonvegan counterpart.

SERVES 6

6 cups vegetable broth

1 carrot, diced

2 ribs celery, diced

1 onion, chopped

½ cup TVP

2 bay leaves

1½ teaspoons Italian seasoning

Salt and pepper, to taste

1 cup vegan noodles or small pasta

Folic Acid: 🖐

Vitamin B$_{12}$: NA

Protein: 🖐

Iron: 🖐

Zinc: 🖐

Calcium: 🖐

Vitamin D: NA

1. Combine all ingredients in a large soup or stockpot.
2. Cover and simmer for 15–20 minutes.

Per Serving
Calories: 123 | Fat: 0g | Sodium: 960mg | Fiber: 3g | Protein: 7g

Black Bean and Butternut Squash Chili

Squash is an excellent addition to vegetarian chili in this Southwestern-style dish.

SERVES 6

1 onion, chopped

3 cloves garlic, minced

2 tablespoons olive oil

1 medium butternut squash, peeled and chopped into chunks

2 (15-ounce) cans black beans, drained and rinsed

1 (28-ounce) can stewed or diced tomatoes, undrained

¾ cup water or vegetable broth

1 tablespoon chili powder

1 teaspoon cumin

¼ teaspoon cayenne pepper, or to taste

½ teaspoon salt, or to taste

2 tablespoons chopped fresh cilantro (optional)

Folic Acid: 🍎🍎🍎

Vitamin B₁₂: NA

Protein: 🍎🍎🍎

Iron: 🍎🍎

Zinc: 🍎

Calcium: 🍎🍎

Vitamin D: NA

1. In a large stockpot, sauté onion and garlic in oil until soft, about 4 minutes.
2. Reduce heat; add remaining ingredients except cilantro. Cover and simmer for 25 minutes.
3. Uncover and simmer another 5 minutes. Top with fresh cilantro just before serving.

Per Serving
Calories: 304 | Fat: 6g | Sodium: 832mg | Fiber: 16g | Protein: 16g

Shiitake and Garlic Broth

Shiitake mushrooms transform ordinary broth into a rich stock with a deep flavor.

YIELDS 6 CUPS

⅓ cup dried shiitake mushrooms

6 cups water

2 cloves garlic, smashed

1 bay leaf

½ teaspoon thyme

½ onion, chopped

Folic Acid: only present in very small amounts

Vitamin B$_{12}$: NA

Protein: only present in very small amounts

Iron: only present in very small amounts

Zinc: only present in very small amounts

Calcium: 🍎

Vitamin D: NA

① In a large soup or stockpot, combine all ingredients; bring to a slow simmer.

② Cover and allow to cook for at least 30–40 minutes.

③ Strain before using.

Per Cup
Calories: 8 | Fat: 0g | Sodium: 5mg | Fiber: 0g | Protein: 0g

Vegetarian Dashi

To turn this into a Japanese dashi stock for miso and noodle soups, omit the bay leaf and thyme and add a generous amount of seaweed, preferably kombu, if you can find it!

African Peanut and Greens Soup

Cut back on the red pepper flakes if you're not a fan of spicy foods, or reduce the liquids to turn it into a thick and chunky curry to pour over rice. Although the ingredients are all familiar, this is definitely not a boring meal!

SERVES 4

1 onion, diced

3 tomatoes, chopped

2 tablespoons olive oil

2 cups vegetable broth

1 cup coconut milk

⅓ cup peanut butter

1 (15-ounce) can chickpeas, drained and rinsed

½ teaspoon salt, or to taste

1 teaspoon curry powder

1 teaspoon sugar

⅛ teaspoon red pepper flakes

1 bunch fresh spinach, stemmed

Folic Acid: 🍎🍎🍎

Vitamin B$_{12}$: NA

Protein: 🍎🍎

Iron: 🍎🍎

Zinc: 🍎🍎

Calcium: 🍎🍎

Vitamin D: NA

1. Sauté the onions and tomatoes in olive oil until onions are soft, about 2–3 minutes.
2. Reduce heat to medium-low; add remaining ingredients except spinach. Stir well to combine.
3. Simmer on low heat, uncovered, stirring occasionally, for 8–10 minutes.
4. Add spinach and allow to cook for another 1–2 minutes, just until spinach is wilted.
5. Remove from heat and adjust seasonings to taste. Soup will thicken as it cools.

Per Serving
Calories: 408 | Fat: 24g | Sodium: 1,202mg | Fiber: 8g | Protein: 13g

Barley Vegetable Soup

Barley Vegetable Soup is an excellent "kitchen sink" recipe, meaning that you can toss in just about any fresh or frozen vegetables or spices you happen to have on hand.

SERVES 6

1 onion, chopped

2 carrots, sliced

2 ribs celery, chopped

2 tablespoons olive oil

8 cups vegetable broth

1 cup barley, uncooked

1½ cups frozen mixed vegetables

1 (14-ounce) can crushed or diced tomatoes

½ teaspoon parsley

½ teaspoon thyme

2 bay leaves

Salt and pepper, to taste

Folic Acid: 🍏

Vitamin B$_{12}$: NA

Protein: 🍏

Iron: 🍏

Zinc: 🍏

Calcium: 🍏

Vitamin D: NA

1. In a large soup or stockpot, sauté the onion, carrots, and celery in olive oil for 3–5 minutes, just until onions are almost soft.
2. Reduce heat to medium-low; add remaining ingredients except salt and pepper.
3. Bring to a simmer; cover, and allow to cook for at least 45 minutes, stirring occasionally.
4. Remove cover; allow to cook for 10 more minutes.
5. Remove bay leaves; season with salt and pepper to taste.

Per Serving
Calories: 228 | Fat: 5g | Sodium: 1,380mg | Fiber: 9g | Protein: 6g

Cream of Carrot Soup with Coconut

This carrot soup will knock your socks off! The addition of coconut milk transforms an ordinary carrot and ginger soup into an unexpected treat.

SERVES 6

3 medium carrots, chopped

1 sweet potato, peeled and chopped

1 yellow onion, chopped

3½ cups vegetable broth

3 cloves garlic, minced

2 teaspoons minced fresh ginger

1 (14-ounce) can coconut milk

1 teaspoon salt, or to taste

¾ teaspoon cinnamon (optional)

Folic Acid: 🍎

Vitamin B$_{12}$: NA

Protein: 🍎

Iron: 🍎

Zinc: 🍎

Calcium: 🍎

Vitamin D: NA

1. In a large soup or stockpot, bring the carrots, sweet potato, and onion to a simmer in the broth.
2. Add garlic and ginger; cover, and heat for 20–25 minutes, until carrots and potatoes are soft.
3. Allow to cool slightly; transfer to a blender, and purée until smooth.
4. Return soup to pot. Over very low heat, stir in the coconut milk and salt, stirring well to combine. Heat just until heated through, another 3–4 minutes.
5. Garnish with cinnamon just before serving.

Per Serving
Calories: 177 | Fat: 14g | Sodium: 978mg | Fiber: 2g | Protein: 2g

Easy Roasted Tomato Soup

Use the freshest, ripest, juiciest red tomatoes you can find for this super-easy recipe, as there are fewer other added flavors. If you find that you need a bit more spice, add a spoonful of nutritional yeast, a dash of cayenne pepper, or an extra shake of salt and pepper.

SERVES 4

6 large tomatoes

1 small onion, peeled

4 cloves garlic, peeled

2 tablespoons olive oil

1¼ cups unflavored fortified soymilk

2 tablespoons chopped fresh basil

1½ teaspoons balsamic vinegar

¾ teaspoon salt, or to taste

¼ teaspoon black pepper

Folic Acid: ♦

Vitamin B₁₂: ♦♦♦

Protein: ♦

Iron: ♦

Zinc: ♦

Calcium: ♦♦

Vitamin D: ♦

1. Preheat oven to 425°F.
2. Slice tomatoes in half and chop onion into quarters. Place tomatoes, onion, and garlic on baking sheet and drizzle with olive oil.
3. Roast in the oven for 45 minutes to 1 hour.
4. Carefully transfer tomatoes, onion, and garlic to a blender, including any juices on the baking sheet. Add remaining ingredients; purée until almost smooth.
5. Reheat over low heat for 1–2 minutes if needed; adjust seasonings to taste.

Per Serving
Calories: 153 | Fat: 9g | Sodium: 488mg | Fiber: 4g | Protein: 5g

Indian Curried Lentil Soup

Similar to a traditional Indian lentil dal recipe, but with added vegetables to make it into an entrée, this lentil soup is perfect as is or paired with rice or some warmed Indian flatbread.

SERVES 4

1 onion, diced

1 carrot, sliced

3 whole cloves

2 tablespoons vegan margarine

1 teaspoon cumin

1 teaspoon turmeric

1 cup yellow or green lentils, uncooked

2¾ cups vegetable broth

2 large tomatoes, chopped

1 teaspoon salt, or to taste

¼ teaspoon black pepper

1 teaspoon lemon juice

Folic Acid: 🍎🍎🍎

Vitamin B₁₂: NA

Protein: 🍎🍎

Iron: 🍎🍎

Zinc: 🍎🍎🍎

Calcium: 🍎

Vitamin D: NA

1. In a large soup or stockpot, sauté the onion, carrot, and cloves in margarine until onions are just turning soft, about 3 minutes. Add cumin and turmeric; toast for 1 minute, stirring constantly to avoid burning.
2. Reduce heat to medium-low; add lentils, broth, tomatoes, and salt. Bring to a simmer; cover, and cook for 35–40 minutes, or until lentils are done.
3. Strain out the cloves. Season with black pepper and lemon juice just before serving.

Per Serving
Calories: 265 | Fat: 6g | Sodium: 1,328mg | Fiber: 17g | Protein: 14g

White Bean and Orzo Minestrone

Italian minestrone is a simple and universally loved soup. This version uses tiny orzo pasta, cannellini beans, and plenty of veggies.

SERVES 6

3 cloves garlic, minced

1 onion, chopped

2 ribs celery, chopped

2 tablespoons olive oil

5 cups vegetable broth

1 carrot, diced

1 cup green beans, chopped

2 small potatoes, chopped small

2 tomatoes, chopped

1 (15-ounce) can cannellini beans, drained and rinsed

1 teaspoon basil

½ teaspoon oregano

¾ cup orzo

Salt and pepper, to taste

Folic Acid: 🍎🍎🍎

Vitamin B$_{12}$: NA

Protein: 🍎🍎

Iron: 🍎🍎🍎

Zinc: 🍎🍎

Calcium: 🍎

Vitamin D: NA

1. In a large soup pot, heat garlic, onion, and celery in olive oil until just soft, about 3–4 minutes.
2. Add broth, carrot, green beans, potatoes, tomatoes, beans, basil, and oregano; bring to a simmer. Cover, and cook on medium-low heat for 20–25 minutes.
3. Add orzo; heat another 10 minutes, just until orzo is cooked. Season well with salt and pepper.

Per Serving
Calories: 304 | Fat: 5g | Sodium: 814mg | Fiber: 8g | Protein: 11g

Ten-Minute Cheater's Chili

No time? No problem! This is a quick and easy way to get some veggies and protein on the table with no hassle. Instead of veggie burgers, you could toss in a handful of TVP flakes, if you'd like, or any other mock meat you happen to have on hand.

SERVES 4

1 (12-ounce) jar salsa

1 (14-ounce) can diced tomatoes

2 (15-ounce) cans kidney beans or black beans, drained and rinsed

1½ cups frozen mixed veggies

4 veggie burgers, crumbled (optional)

2 tablespoons chili powder

1 teaspoon cumin

½ cup water

Folic Acid: 🍎🍎

Vitamin B$_{12}$: NA

Protein: 🍎🍎

Iron: 🍎🍎🍎

Zinc: 🍎🍎

Calcium: 🍎🍎

Vitamin D: NA

① In a large pot, combine all ingredients.
② Simmer for 10 minutes, stirring frequently.

Per Serving
Calories: 271 | Fat: 3g | Sodium: 1,154mg | Fiber: 17g | Protein: 15g

Thai Tom Kha Coconut Soup

In Thailand, this soup is a full meal, served alongside a large plate of steamed rice. Don't worry if you can't find lemongrass or galangal, as lime and ginger add a similar flavor.

SERVES 4

1 (14-ounce) can coconut milk

2 cups vegetable broth

1 tablespoon soy sauce

3 cloves garlic, minced

5 slices fresh ginger or galangal

1 stalk lemongrass, chopped (optional)

1 tablespoon lime juice

1–2 small chilies, chopped

½ teaspoon red pepper flakes, or to taste

1 onion, chopped

2 tomatoes, chopped

1 carrot, sliced thin

½ cup sliced mushrooms, any kind

¼ cup chopped fresh cilantro

Folic Acid: 🍎

Vitamin B$_{12}$: NA

Protein: 🍎

Iron: 🍎🍎

Zinc: 🍎

Calcium: 🍎

Vitamin D: only present in very small amounts

1. Over medium-low heat, combine the coconut milk and vegetable broth. Add soy sauce, garlic, ginger, lemongrass, lime juice, chilies, and red pepper flakes; heat for about 10 minutes, but do not boil.
2. When broth is hot, add onion, tomatoes, carrot, and mushrooms. Cover, and cook on low heat for 10–15 minutes.
3. Remove from heat; top with chopped fresh cilantro.

Per Serving
Calories: 240 | Fat: 21g | Sodium: 725mg | Fiber: 2g | Protein: 4g

Cold Spanish Gazpacho with Avocado

This soup is best enjoyed on an outdoor patio just after sunset on a warm summer evening. But really, anytime you want a simple light starter soup will do, no matter the weather. Add some crunch by topping with home-made croutons.

SERVES 6

2 cucumbers, diced

½ red onion, diced

2 large tomatoes, diced

¼ cup fresh chopped cilantro

2 avocados, diced

4 cloves garlic

2 tablespoons lime juice

1 tablespoon red wine vinegar

¾ cup vegetable broth

1 chili pepper (jalapeño, serrano, or cayenne) or 1 teaspoon hot sauce

Salt and pepper, to taste

Folic Acid: 🍎 🍎

Vitamin B$_{12}$: NA

Protein: 🍎

Iron: 🍎

Zinc: 🍎

Calcium: 🍎

Vitamin D: NA

1. Mix together the cucumbers, red onion, tomatoes, cilantro, and avocado. Set half of the mixture aside.
2. In a blender, mix the other half of the vegetable mixture. Add the garlic, lime juice, vinegar, vegetable broth, and chili pepper; process until smooth.
3. Transfer to serving bowl; add remaining diced cucumbers, onion, tomatoes, cilantro, and avocado, stirring gently to combine.
4. Season with salt and pepper, to taste.

Per Serving
Calories: 149 | Fat: 10g | Sodium: 130mg | Fiber: 7g | Protein: 3g

Kidney Bean and Zucchini Gumbo

This vegetable gumbo uses zucchini instead of okra. Traditional gumbo always calls for ground sassafras leaves, known as filé powder. If you can't find this anywhere, increase the amounts of the other spices.

SERVES 5

1 onion, diced

1 red or green bell pepper, chopped

3 ribs celery, chopped

2 tablespoons olive oil

1 zucchini, sliced

1 (14-ounce) can diced tomatoes

3 cups vegetable broth

1 teaspoon hot sauce

1 teaspoon filé powder (optional)

¾ teaspoon thyme

1 teaspoon Cajun seasoning

2 bay leaves

1 (15-ounce) can kidney beans, drained and rinsed

1½ cups cooked rice

Folic Acid: 🍎🍎

Vitamin B$_{12}$: NA

Protein: 🍎

Iron: 🍎🍎

Zinc: 🍎

Calcium: 🍎

Vitamin D: NA

1. In a large soup or stockpot, sauté the onion, bell pepper, and celery in olive oil for 1–2 minutes. Reduce heat; add remaining ingredients, except beans and rice.
2. Bring to a simmer; cover, and allow to cook for 30 minutes.
3. Uncover; add beans, and stir to combine. Heat for 5 more minutes.
4. Remove bay leaves before serving. Serve over cooked rice.

Per Serving
Calories: 227 | Fat: 6g | Sodium: 1,128mg | Fiber: 7g | Protein: 7g

Potato and Leek Soup

With simple earthy flavors, this classic recipe makes a comforting meal.

SERVES 6

1 yellow onion, diced

2 cloves garlic, minced

2 tablespoons olive oil

6 cups vegetable broth

3 leeks, sliced

2 large potatoes, chopped

2 bay leaves

1 cup unflavored fortified soymilk

2 tablespoons vegan margarine

¾ teaspoon salt, or to taste

⅓ teaspoon black pepper

½ teaspoon sage

½ teaspoon thyme

2 tablespoons nutritional yeast (optional)

Folic Acid: 🍏

Vitamin B₁₂: 🍏

Protein: 🍏

Iron: 🍏

Zinc: 🍏

Calcium: 🍏

Vitamin D: 🍏

1. Sauté onions and garlic in olive oil for 1–2 minutes, until onions are soft.
2. Add broth, leeks, potatoes, and bay leaves; bring to a slow simmer. Cook, partially covered, for 30 minutes, until potatoes are soft.
3. Remove bay leaves. Working in batches as needed, purée soup in a blender until almost smooth, or desired consistency.
4. Return soup to pot; stir in remaining ingredients. Adjust seasonings; reheat as needed.

Per Serving
Calories: 223 | Fat: 9g | Sodium: 1,321mg | Fiber: 4g | Protein: 4g

Cannellini Bean and Corn Chowder

This is a filling and textured soup that could easily be a main dish. Some chopped collards or a dash of hot sauce would be a welcome addition. For a lower fat version, skip the initial sauté and add about 5 minutes to the cooking time.

SERVES 4

1 potato, chopped small

1 onion, chopped

2 tablespoons olive oil

3 cups vegetable broth

2 ears of corn, kernels cut off, or 1½ cups frozen or canned corn

1 (15-ounce) can cannellini or great Northern beans, drained and rinsed

½ teaspoon thyme

¼ teaspoon black pepper

1 tablespoon flour

1½ cups unflavored fortified soymilk

Folic Acid: 🍏🍏

Vitamin B$_{12}$: 🍏🍏🍏

Protein: 🍏🍏

Iron: 🍏🍏

Zinc: 🍏🍏

Calcium: 🍏🍏🍏

Vitamin D: 🍏

1. In a large soup or stockpot, sauté potato and onion in olive oil for 3–5 minutes.
2. Reduce heat and add vegetable broth. Bring to a slow simmer; cover, and allow to cook for 15–20 minutes.
3. Uncover; add corn, beans, thyme, and pepper.
4. Whisk together flour and soymilk; add to the pot, stirring well to prevent lumps.
5. Reduce heat to prevent soymilk from curdling; cook, uncovered, for 5–6 more minutes, stirring frequently.
6. Allow to cool slightly before serving, as soup will thicken as it cools.

Per Serving
Calories: 322 | Fat: 9g | Sodium: 761mg | Fiber: 8g | Protein: 13g

Chinese Hot and Sour Soup

If you can't get enough of old Jackie Chan flicks and Wong Kar-wai films, then this traditional Chinese soup is for you.

SERVES 6

2 cups diced seitan, or other meat substitute

2 tablespoons vegetable oil

1½ teaspoons hot sauce

6 cups vegetable broth

½ head Napa cabbage, shredded

¾ cup sliced shiitake mushrooms

1 (8-ounce) can bamboo shoots, drained

2 tablespoons soy sauce

2 tablespoons white vinegar

¾ teaspoon crushed red pepper flakes

¾ teaspoon salt, or to taste

2 tablespoons cornstarch

¼ cup water

3 scallions, sliced

2 teaspoons sesame oil

Folic Acid: 🍎🍎

Vitamin B₁₂: NA

Protein: 🍎🍎🍎

Iron: 🍎

Zinc: 🍎

Calcium: 🍎

Vitamin D: NA

1. Brown seitan in vegetable oil for 2–3 minutes, until cooked. Reduce heat to low; add hot sauce, stirring well to coat. Cook over low heat for 1 more minute; remove from heat and set aside.
2. In a large soup or stockpot, combine broth, cabbage, mushrooms, bamboo, soy sauce, vinegar, red pepper flakes, and salt. Bring to a slow simmer and cover. Simmer for at least 15 minutes.
3. In a separate small bowl, whisk together the cornstarch and water; slowly stir into soup. Heat just until soup thickens, about 3–5 minutes.
4. Portion into serving bowls; top each serving with scallions and drizzle with sesame oil.

Per Serving
Calories: 195 | Fat: 7g | Sodium: 1,927mg | Fiber: 3g | Protein: 18g

Curried Pumpkin Soup

You don't have to wait for fall to make this pumpkin soup, as canned pumpkin purée will work just fine. It's also excellent with coconut milk instead of soymilk.

SERVES 4

1 yellow onion, diced

3 cloves garlic, minced

2 tablespoons vegan margarine

1 (15-ounce) can pumpkin purée

3 cups vegetable broth

2 bay leaves

1 tablespoon curry powder

1 teaspoon cumin

½ teaspoon ground ginger

1 cup unflavored fortified soymilk

¼ teaspoon salt, or to taste

Folic Acid: 🍎

Vitamin B$_{12}$: 🍎🍎🍎

Protein: 🍎

Iron: 🍎

Zinc: 🍎

Calcium: 🍎🍎

Vitamin D: 🍎

1. In a large soup or stockpot, heat onion and garlic in margarine until onion is soft, about 4–5 minutes.
2. Add pumpkin and broth; stir well to combine. Add bay leaves, curry, cumin, and ginger; bring to a slow simmer.
3. Cover and allow to cook for 15 minutes.
4. Reduce heat to low; add soymilk, stirring to combine. Heat for 1–2 minutes, or until heated through.
5. Season with salt, to taste; remove bay leaves before serving.

Per Serving
Calories: 136 | Fat: 7g | Sodium: 1,112mg | Fiber: 4g | Protein: 3g

Super "Meaty" Chili with TVP

Any mock meat will work well in a vegetarian chili, but TVP is easy to keep on hand and very inexpensive. This is more of a thick, "meaty" Texas chili than a vegetable chili, but chili is easy and forgiving, so if you want to toss in some zucchini, broccoli, or diced carrots, by all means, do!

SERVES 6

1½ cups TVP granules

1 cup hot vegetable broth

1 tablespoon soy sauce

1 yellow onion, chopped

5 cloves garlic, minced

2 tablespoons olive oil

1 cup corn kernels, fresh, frozen, or canned

1 bell pepper, any color, chopped

2 (15-ounce) cans black, kidney, or pinto beans, drained and rinsed

1 (14-ounce) can diced tomatoes

1 jalapeño pepper, minced, or ½ teaspoon cayenne pepper (optional)

1 teaspoon cumin

2 tablespoons chili powder

Salt and pepper, to taste

Folic Acid: 🍎🍎🍎

Vitamin B₁₂: NA

Protein: 🍎🍎🍎

Iron: 🍎🍎

Zinc: 🍎🍎

Calcium: 🍎

Vitamin D: NA

1. Cover the TVP with hot broth and soy sauce. Allow to sit for 3–4 minutes only, then drain.
2. In a large soup or stockpot, sauté the onion and garlic in olive oil until onions are soft, about 3–4 minutes.
3. Add remaining ingredients and TVP, stirring well to combine.
4. Cover, and allow to simmer over low heat for at least 30 minutes, stirring occasionally. Adjust seasonings to taste.

Per Serving
Calories: 272 | Fat: 6g | Sodium: 603mg | Fiber: 13g | Protein: 20g

Udon Noodle Buddha Bowl

This is a nutritious full meal in a bowl, which might be particularly comforting on the edge of a cold or after an early morning meditation. For an authentic Japanese flavor, add a large piece of kombu seaweed to the broth.

SERVES 4

2 (8-ounce) packages udon noodles

3½ cups Shiitake and Garlic Broth (see recipe in this chapter)

1½ teaspoons fresh minced ginger

1 tablespoon sugar

1 tablespoon soy sauce

1 tablespoon rice vinegar

¼ teaspoon red pepper flakes, or to taste

1 baby bok choy, sliced

1 cup mushrooms, any kind, sliced

1 (12-ounce) block silken tofu, cubed

¼ cup bean sprouts

1 cup fresh spinach

1 teaspoon sesame oil or hot chili oil

Folic Acid: 🍎

Vitamin B$_{12}$: NA

Protein: 🍎 🍎

Iron: 🍎

Zinc: 🍎

Calcium: 🍎

Vitamin D: only present in very small amounts

1. Cook noodles in boiling water until soft, about 5 minutes. Drain and divide into 4 serving bowls; set aside.
2. In a large pot, combine the Shiitake and Garlic Broth, ginger, sugar, soy sauce, vinegar, and red pepper flakes; bring to a simmer.
3. Add bok choy, mushrooms, and tofu; cook just until veggies are soft, about 10 minutes.
4. Add bean sprouts and spinach; simmer for 1 more minute, until spinach has wilted.
5. Remove from heat; drizzle with sesame oil or chili oil.
6. Divide soup into the 4 bowls containing cooked noodles; serve immediately.

Per Serving
Calories: 240 | Fat: 4g | Sodium: 453mg | Fiber: 1g | Protein: 12g

Winter Seitan Stew

If you're used to a "meat and potatoes" kind of diet, this hearty seitan and potato stew ought to become a favorite.

SERVES 6

2 cups chopped seitan

1 onion, chopped

2 carrots, chopped

2 ribs celery, chopped

2 tablespoons olive oil

4 cups vegetable broth

2 potatoes, chopped

½ teaspoon sage

½ teaspoon rosemary

½ teaspoon thyme

2 tablespoons cornstarch

⅓ cup water

Salt and pepper, to taste

Folic Acid: 🍎

Vitamin B$_{12}$: NA

Protein: 🍎🍎🍎

Iron: 🍎

Zinc: 🍎

Calcium: 🍎

Vitamin D: NA

1. In a large soup pot, heat seitan, onion, carrots, and celery in olive oil for 4–5 minutes, stirring frequently, until seitan is lightly browned.
2. Add vegetable broth and potatoes; bring to a boil.
3. Reduce to a simmer; add spices, and cover. Allow to cook for 25–30 minutes, until potatoes are soft.
4. In a small bowl, whisk together cornstarch and water. Add to soup; stir to combine.
5. Cook, uncovered, for another 5–7 minutes, until stew has thickened.
6. Season with salt and pepper, to taste.

Per Serving
Calories: 213 | Fat: 6g | Sodium: 974mg | Fiber: 4g | Protein: 17g

Cashew Cream of Asparagus Soup

A dairy-free and soy-free asparagus soup with a rich cashew base brings out the natural flavors of the asparagus without relying on other enhancers.

SERVES 4

1 onion, chopped

4 cloves garlic, minced

2 tablespoons olive oil

2 pounds asparagus, trimmed and chopped

4 cups vegetable broth

¾ cup raw cashews

¾ cup water

¼ teaspoon sage

½ teaspoon salt

¼ teaspoon black pepper

2 teaspoons lemon juice

2 tablespoons nutritional yeast

Folic Acid: 🍎🍎🍎

Vitamin B₁₂: 🍎🍎🍎

Protein: 🍎🍎

Iron: 🍎🍎🍎

Zinc: 🍎🍎🍎

Calcium: 🍎

Vitamin D: NA

1. In a large soup or stockpot, sauté onion and garlic in olive oil for 2–3 minutes until onion is soft. Reduce heat and carefully add asparagus and vegetable broth.
2. Bring to a simmer, cover, and cook for 20 minutes. Cool slightly, then purée in a blender, working in batches as needed until almost smooth. Return to pot over low heat.
3. Purée together cashews and water until smooth and add to soup. Add sage, salt, and pepper and heat for a few more minutes, stirring to combine.
4. Stir in lemon juice and nutritional yeast just before serving, and adjust seasonings to taste.

Per Serving
Calories: 284 | Fat: 18g | Sodium: 1,242mg | Fiber: 7g | Protein: 11g

Garlic Miso and Onion Soup

Boiling miso destroys some of its beneficial enzymes, so be sure to heat this soup to just below a simmer. Use a soft hand when slicing the silken tofu, so it doesn't crumble.

SERVES 4

5 cups water

½ cup sliced shiitake mushrooms

3 scallions, chopped

½ onion, chopped

4 cloves garlic, minced

¾ teaspoon garlic powder

2 tablespoons soy sauce

1 teaspoon sesame oil

1 (12-ounce) block silken tofu, diced

⅓ cup miso

1 tablespoon chopped seaweed, any kind (optional)

Folic Acid: 🍎

Vitamin B$_{12}$: NA

Protein: 🍎🍎

Iron: 🍎

Zinc: 🍎🍎

Calcium: 🍎

Vitamin D: only present in very small amounts

1. Combine all ingredients except for miso and seaweed in a large soup or stockpot and bring to a slow simmer. Cook, uncovered, for 10–12 minutes.
2. Reduce heat and stir in miso and seaweed, being careful not to boil.
3. Heat, stirring to dissolve miso, for another 5 minutes until onions and mushrooms are soft.

Per Serving
Calories: 133 | Fat: 5g | Sodium: 1,336mg | Fiber: 2g | Protein: 10g

Vegan Cream Cheese and Butternut Squash Soup

This isn't a healthy, hippie vegetable soup—it's a rich, decadent, stick-to-your-thighs soup. Nonetheless, it's absolutely delicious. Top with a mountain of homemade croutons or serve with crusty French bread.

SERVES 4

2 cloves garlic, minced

½ yellow onion, diced

2 tablespoons olive oil

3½ cups vegetable broth

1 medium butternut squash, peeled, seeded, and chopped into cubes

1 teaspoon curry powder

¼ teaspoon nutmeg

½ (8-ounce) container vegan cream cheese

¼ teaspoon salt

Folic Acid: 🍏

Vitamin B$_{12}$: NA

Protein: 🍏

Iron: 🍏

Zinc: 🍏

Calcium: 🍏

Vitamin D: NA

1. In a large skillet or stockpot, sauté garlic and onion in olive oil until soft, about 3–4 minutes.
2. Reduce heat to medium-low and add vegetable broth, squash, curry powder, and nutmeg. Simmer for 25 minutes until squash is soft.
3. Working in batches, purée until almost smooth, or to desired consistency. Or, if squash is soft enough, mash smooth with a large fork.
4. Return soup to very low heat and stir in vegan cream cheese until melted, combined, and heated through. Add salt and adjust seasonings to taste.

Per Serving
Calories: 212 | Fat: 12g | Sodium: 1,133mg | Fiber: 3g | Protein: 2g

CHAPTER 9

Desserts

Strawberry Coconut Ice Cream

Rich and creamy, this is the most decadent dairy-free strawberry ice cream you'll ever taste.

SERVES 6

2 cups coconut cream

1¾ cups frozen strawberries

¾ cup sugar

2 teaspoons vanilla

¼ teaspoon salt

Folic Acid: 🍏

Vitamin B₁₂: NA

Protein: 🍏

Iron: 🍏

Zinc: 🍏

Calcium: only present in very small amounts

Vitamin D: NA

① Purée together all ingredients until smooth and creamy.

② Transfer mixture to a large freezer-proof baking or casserole dish; freeze.

③ Stir every 30 minutes, until a smooth ice cream forms, about 4 hours. If mixture gets too firm, transfer to a blender, process until smooth, then return to freezer.

Per Serving
Calories: 475 | Fat: 16g | Sodium: 134mg | Fiber: 2g | Protein: 1g

Vegan Chocolate Hazelnut Spread

Treat yourself with this rich, sticky chocolate spread. This one will have you dancing around the kitchen and licking your spoons!

YIELDS 1 CUP

2 cups hazelnuts, chopped
½ cup cocoa powder
¾ cup powdered sugar
½ teaspoon vanilla
4–5 tablespoons vegetable oil

Folic Acid: 🍎
Vitamin B$_{12}$: NA
Protein: 🍎
Iron: 🍎
Zinc: 🍎
Calcium: 🍎
Vitamin D: NA

1. In a food processor, process hazelnuts until very finely ground, about 3–4 minutes.
2. Add cocoa powder, sugar, and vanilla; process to combine.
3. Add oil, a little bit at a time, until mixture is soft and creamy and desired consistency is reached. You may need to add a bit more or less than 4–5 tablespoons.

Per Tablespoon
Calories: 164 | Fat: 14g | Sodium: 1mg | Fiber: 3g | Protein: 3g

Apricot Ginger Sorbet

Made with real fruit and without dairy, this is a nearly fat-free treat that you can add to smoothies or just enjoy outside on a hot summer day.

SERVES 6

⅔ cup water

⅔ cup sugar

2 teaspoons fresh minced ginger

5 cups chopped apricots, fresh or frozen

3 tablespoons lemon juice

Folic Acid: 🍏

Vitamin B₁₂: NA

Protein: 🍏

Iron: 🍏

Zinc: 🍏

Calcium: 🍏

Vitamin D: NA

① Bring the water, sugar, and ginger to a boil; reduce to a slow simmer. Heat for 3–4 more minutes, until sugar is dissolved and a syrup forms. Allow to cool.

② Purée the sugar syrup, apricots, and lemon juice until smooth.

③ Transfer mixture to a large freezer-proof baking or casserole dish; freeze.

④ Stir every 30 minutes, until a smooth ice cream forms, about 4 hours. If mixture gets too firm, transfer to a blender, process until smooth, then return to freezer.

Per Serving
Calories: 154 | Fat: 1g | Sodium: 2mg | Fiber: 3g | Protein: 2g

Chocolate Peanut Butter Pudding

Whoever first combined chocolate and peanut butter deserves a Nobel Prize. Or at least a MacArthur "Genius Grant."

SERVES 4

1 (12-ounce) block silken tofu

¼ cup cocoa powder

½ teaspoon vanilla

¼ cup peanut butter or other nut butter

¼ cup maple syrup or brown rice syrup

Folic Acid: only present in very small amounts

Vitamin B₁₂: NA

Protein: 🍎🍎

Iron: 🍎

Zinc: 🍎

Calcium: 🍎

Vitamin D: NA

- Process all ingredients together until smooth and creamy.

Per Serving
Calories: 213 | Fat: 11g | Sodium: 110mg | Fiber: 3g | Protein: 10g

Coconut Rice Pudding

The combination of juicy soft mango with tropical coconut milk is simply heavenly, but if mangos are unavailable, pineapples or strawberries would add a delicious touch to this refined lightly sweetened dessert.

SERVES 4

1½ cups cooked white rice

1½ cups fortified vanilla soymilk

1½ cups coconut milk

3 tablespoons brown rice syrup or maple syrup

2 tablespoons agave nectar

4-5 dates, chopped

Dash cinnamon or nutmeg

2 mangos, chopped

Folic Acid: 🍎🍎

Vitamin B₁₂: 🍎🍎🍎

Protein: 🍎

Iron: 🍎🍎

Zinc: 🍎🍎

Calcium: 🍎🍎

Vitamin D: 🍎

1. Combine rice, soymilk, and coconut milk over low heat. Bring to a very low simmer for 10 minutes, or until mixture starts to thicken.
2. Stir in brown rice syrup, agave nectar, and dates; heat for another 2–3 minutes.
3. Allow to cool slightly before serving to allow pudding to thicken slightly. Garnish with a dash of cinnamon and fresh fruit just before serving.

Per Serving
Calories: 448 | Fat: 20g | Sodium: 51mg | Fiber: 3g | Protein: 6g

Easy Banana Date Cookies

Once you hit your third trimester, anything easy sounds pretty perfect. However, these Easy Banana Date Cookies are delicious any time the craving hits!

YIELDS 1 DOZEN COOKIES

1 cup chopped pitted dates

1 banana, medium ripe

¼ teaspoon vanilla

1¾ cups coconut flakes

Folic Acid: only present in very small amounts

Vitamin B$_{12}$: NA

Protein: 🍎

Iron: only present in very small amounts

Zinc: 🍎

Calcium: only present in very small amounts

Vitamin D: NA

1. Preheat oven to 375°F. Cover dates in water and soak for about 10 minutes, until softened. Drain.
2. Process the dates, banana, and vanilla until almost smooth. Stir in coconut flakes by hand until thick. You may need a little more or less than 1¾ cups.
3. Drop by generous tablespoonfuls onto a cookie sheet. Bake 10–12 minutes, or until done. Cookies will be soft and chewy.

Per Cookie
Calories: 111 | Fat: 6g | Sodium: 4mg | Fiber: 3g | Protein: 1g

Chocolate Mocha Ice Cream

If you have an ice-cream maker, you can skip the stirring and freezing and just add the blended ingredients to your machine.

SERVES 6

1 cup vegan chocolate chips

1 cup fortified soymilk

1 (12-ounce) block silken tofu

⅓ cup sugar

2 tablespoons instant coffee

2 teaspoons vanilla

¼ teaspoon salt

Folic Acid: only present in very small amounts

Vitamin B$_{12}$: 🍎🍎

Protein: 🍎

Iron: 🍎

Zinc: 🍎

Calcium: 🍎

Vitamin D: 🍎

1. Using a double broiler, or over very low heat, melt chocolate chips until smooth and creamy, about 5 minutes. Allow to cool slightly.
2. Blend together the soymilk, tofu, sugar, coffee, vanilla, and salt until smooth, at least 2 minutes.
3. Add melted chocolate chips; process until smooth.
4. Transfer mixture to a large freezer-proof baking or casserole dish; freeze.
5. Stir every 30 minutes, until a smooth ice cream forms, about 4 hours. If mixture gets too firm, transfer to a blender, process until smooth, then return to freezer.

Per Serving
Calories: 150 | Fat: 8g | Sodium: 120mg | Fiber: 0g | Protein: 5g

No-Bake Cocoa Balls

Craving a healthy chocolate snack? Try these fudgy little cocoa balls, similar to a soft no-bake cookie, but with no refined sugar.

SERVES 4

1 cup chopped pitted dates

1 cup walnuts or cashews

¼ cup cocoa powder

1 tablespoon peanut butter

¼ cup coconut flakes

Folic Acid: 🍎

Vitamin B$_{12}$: NA

Protein: 🍎

Iron: 🍎

Zinc: 🍎 🍎

Calcium: 🍎

Vitamin D: NA

1. Cover dates in water; soak for about 10 minutes, until softened. Drain.
2. In a food processor, process dates, nuts, cocoa powder, and peanut butter until combined and sticky.
3. Add coconut flakes; process until coarse.
4. Shape into balls; chill.
5. If mixture is too wet, add more nuts and coconut; add just a touch of water if the mixture is dry and crumbly.

Per Serving
Calories: 348 | Fat: 22g | Sodium: 23mg | Fiber: 8g | Protein: 7g

Variations

Roll these little balls in extra coconut flakes for a sweet presentation, or try it with carob powder instead of cocoa—they're just as satisfying. Don't have fresh dates on hand? Raisins may be substituted, but skip the soaking. Even with raisins, you really won't believe they're sugar free.

Chewy Oatmeal Raisin Cookies

The addition of applesauce keeps these classic nostalgic cookies super chewy. No egg replacer needed!

YIELDS 1½ DOZEN COOKIES

⅓ cup vegan margarine, softened

½ cup brown sugar

¼ cup granulated sugar

⅓ cup applesauce

1 teaspoon vanilla

2 tablespoons fortified soymilk

¾ cup whole-wheat flour

½ teaspoon baking soda

½ teaspoon cinnamon

½ teaspoon ginger

1¾ cups quick-cooking oats

⅔ cup raisins

Folic Acid: only present in very small amounts

Vitamin B$_{12}$: NA

Protein: 🍎

Iron: 🍎

Zinc: 🍎

Calcium: only present in very small amounts

Vitamin D: only present in very small amounts

1. Preheat oven to 350°F.
2. Beat the margarine and sugars together until smooth and creamy. Add applesauce, vanilla, and soymilk.
3. Sift together the flour, baking soda, cinnamon, and ginger; add to wet ingredients.
4. Stir in oats, then raisins; drop by generous spoonfuls onto a cookie sheet.
5. Bake for 10–12 minutes, or until done.

Per Cookie
Calories: 122 | Fat: 4g | Sodium: 85mg | Fiber: 2g | Protein: 2g

Quinoa "Tapioca" Pudding

Instead of tapioca pudding or baked rice pudding, try this whole-grain version made with quinoa. Healthy enough to eat for breakfast, but sweet enough for dessert, too.

SERVES 4

1 cup quinoa

2 cups water

2 cups fortified soymilk or soy creamer

2 tablespoons maple syrup or brown rice syrup

1 teaspoon cornstarch

2 bananas, sliced thin

½ teaspoon vanilla

⅓ cup raisins

Dash cinnamon or nutmeg (optional)

Folic Acid: 🍎🍎

Vitamin B$_{12}$: 🍎🍎🍎

Protein: 🍎🍎

Iron: 🍎🍎

Zinc: 🍎🍎

Calcium: 🍎🍎

Vitamin D: 🍎

1. In a medium saucepan over medium heat, simmer quinoa in water, covered, stirring frequently, for 10–15 minutes, until done and water is absorbed.
2. Reduce heat to medium-low. Stir in soymilk, maple syrup, cornstarch, and bananas; combine well.
3. Heat, stirring constantly, for 6–8 minutes, until bananas are soft and pudding has thickened.
4. Stir in vanilla and raisins while still hot; sprinkle with a dash of cinnamon, to taste.

Per Serving
Calories: 325 | Fat: 5g | Sodium: 67mg | Fiber: 5g | Protein: 11g

Pumpkin Maple Pie

For Thanksgiving or any time, this pie supplies plenty of vitamin A from the pumpkin.

SERVES 8

1 (16-ounce) can pumpkin purée

½ cup maple syrup

1 (12-ounce) block silken tofu

¼ cup sugar

1½ teaspoons cinnamon

½ teaspoon ginger powder

½ teaspoon nutmeg

¼ teaspoon ground cloves (optional)

½ teaspoon salt

1 vegan prepared pie crust

Folic Acid: only present in very small amounts

Vitamin B$_{12}$: NA

Protein: 🍎

Iron: 🍎

Zinc: 🍎🍎

Calcium: 🍎

Vitamin D: NA

1. Preheat oven to 400°F.
2. In a blender or food processor, process the pumpkin, maple syrup, and tofu until smooth and creamy.
3. Add sugar and spices; pour into pie crust.
4. Bake for 1 hour, or until done. Allow to cool before slicing and serving, as pie will set and firm as it cools.

Per Serving
Calories: 266 | Fat: 9g | Sodium: 381mg | Fiber: 2g | Protein: 3g

Classic Chocolate Chip Cookies

Just like mom used to make, only with a little applesauce to cut down on the fat a bit.

YIELDS ABOUT 2 DOZEN COOKIES

⅔ cup vegan margarine

⅔ cup granulated sugar

⅔ cup brown sugar

⅓ cup applesauce

1½ teaspoons vanilla

Egg replacer for 2 eggs

2½ cups flour

1 teaspoon baking soda

½ teaspoon baking powder

1 teaspoon salt

⅔ cup quick-cooking oats

1½ cups vegan chocolate chips

Folic Acid: 🍎

Vitamin B₁₂: NA

Protein: 🍎

Iron: 🍎

Zinc: 🍎

Calcium: 🍎

Vitamin D: NA

1. Preheat oven to 375°F.
2. In a large mixing bowl, cream together the margarine and granulated sugar; mix in brown sugar, applesauce, vanilla, and egg replacer.
3. In a separate bowl, combine the flour, baking soda, baking powder, and salt; combine with the wet ingredients. Mix well.
4. Stir in oats and chocolate chips just until combined.
5. Drop by generous spoonfuls onto a baking sheet; bake for 10–12 minutes.

Per Cookie
Calories: 161 | Fat: 7g | Sodium: 232mg | Fiber: 1g | Protein: 2g

Maple Date Carrot Cake

With applesauce for moisture and just a touch of oil, this is a cake you can feel good about eating for breakfast. Leave out the dates if you want even less natural sugar.

SERVES 8

1½ cups raisins

1⅓ cups pineapple juice

6 dates, diced

2¼ cups grated carrot

½ cup maple syrup

¼ cup applesauce

2 tablespoons oil

3 cups flour

1½ teaspoons baking soda

½ teaspoon salt

1 teaspoon cinnamon

½ teaspoon allspice or nutmeg

Egg replacer for 2 eggs

Folic Acid: 🍎🍎

Vitamin B$_{12}$: NA

Protein: 🍎

Iron: 🍎🍎

Zinc: 🍎🍎

Calcium: 🍎

Vitamin D: NA

1. Preheat oven to 375°F; grease and flour a cake pan.
2. Combine the raisins with pineapple juice; allow to sit for 5–10 minutes to soften.
3. In a separate small bowl, cover the dates with water until soft, about 10 minutes. Drain water.
4. In a large mixing bowl, combine the raisins and pineapple juice, carrot, maple syrup, applesauce, oil, and dates.
5. In a separate large bowl, combine the flour, baking soda, salt, cinnamon, and allspice.
6. Combine the dry ingredients with the wet ingredients; add prepared egg replacer. Mix well.
7. Pour batter into prepared cake pan; bake for 30 minutes, or until a toothpick inserted in the center comes out clean.

Per Serving
Calories: 394 | Fat: 4g | Sodium: 406mg | Fiber: 4g | Protein: 6g

Sweetheart Raspberry Lemon Cupcakes

Add ½ teaspoon of lemon extract for extra lemony goodness in these sweet and tart cupcakes. Or omit the raspberries and add 3 tablespoons of poppy seeds for lemon poppy seed cupcakes. These sweets are amazing any way you cut it!

YIELDS 18 CUPCAKES

½ cup vegan margarine, softened

1 cup sugar

½ teaspoon vanilla

⅔ cup fortified soymilk

3 tablespoons lemon juice

Zest from 2 lemons

1¾ cups flour

1½ teaspoons baking powder

½ teaspoon baking soda

¼ teaspoon salt

¾ cup diced raspberries, fresh or frozen

Folic Acid: 🍎

Vitamin B$_{12}$: 🍎

Protein: 🍎

Iron: 🍎

Zinc: only present in very small amounts

Calcium: 🍎

Vitamin D: only present in very small amounts

1. Preheat oven to 350°F; grease or line a cupcake tin.
2. Beat together the margarine and sugar until light and fluffy.
3. Add vanilla, soymilk, lemon juice, and zest.
4. In a separate bowl, sift together the flour, baking powder, baking soda, and salt.
5. Combine flour mixture with wet ingredients just until mixed; do not overmix.
6. Gently fold in diced raspberries.
7. Fill cupcakes about two-thirds full with batter; bake immediately for 16–18 minutes, or until done.

Per Cupcake
Calories: 139 | Fat: 5g | Sodium: 182mg | Fiber: 1g | Protein: 2g

Raspberry Cream Cheese Frosting

Combine half an 8-ounce container of vegan cream cheese with ½ cup raspberry jam and 6 tablespoons of softened vegan margarine. Beat until smooth, then add powdered sugar until a creamy frosting forms. You'll need about 2½ cups. Pile it high and garnish your cupcakes with fresh strawberry slices or pink vegan candies.

Foolproof Vegan Fudge

Vegan fudge is much easier to make than nonvegan fudge, so don't worry about a thing when making this recipe. Regular soymilk will work just fine, but soy creamer has a richer taste.

YIELDS 24 1" PIECES

⅓ cup vegan margarine

⅓ cup cocoa

⅓ cup soy creamer

½ teaspoon vanilla

2 tablespoons peanut butter

3–3½ cups powdered sugar

¾ cup nuts, finely chopped

Folic Acid: only present in very small amounts

Vitamin B$_{12}$: NA

Protein: 🍎

Iron: 🍎

Zinc: 🍎

Calcium: only present in very small amounts

Vitamin D: NA

1. Lightly grease a small baking dish or square cake pan.
2. Using a double broiler, or over very low heat, melt the vegan margarine with the cocoa, soy creamer, vanilla, and peanut butter.
3. Slowly incorporate powdered sugar until mixture is smooth, creamy, and thick. Stir in nuts.
4. Immediately transfer to pan and chill until completely firm, at least 2 hours.

Per 2-Piece Serving
Calories: 237 | Fat: 12g | Sodium: 89mg | Fiber: 1g | Protein: 2g

Mint Fudge? Almond Fudge?

For a variation, halve the vanilla extract and add ¼ teaspoon of flavored extract: almond, mint, or whatever you enjoy.

Cocoa-Nut-Coconut No-Bake Cookies

Shape these into little balls, and try not to eat them all along the way!

YIELDS 2 DOZEN COOKIES

¼ cup vegan margarine

½ cup fortified soymilk

2 cups sugar

⅓ cup cocoa

½ cup peanut butter (or other nut butter)

½ teaspoon vanilla

3 cups quick-cooking oats

½ cup walnuts or cashews, finely chopped

½ cup coconut flakes

Folic Acid: 🍎

Vitamin B$_{12}$: 🍎 🍎

Protein: 🍎

Iron: 🍎

Zinc: 🍎

Calcium: only present in very small amounts

Vitamin D: only present in very small amounts

1. Line a baking sheet with wax paper.
2. In a large pot, melt the vegan margarine and soymilk together and add sugar and cocoa. Bring to a quick boil to dissolve sugar, then reduce heat to low and stir in peanut
butter, just until melted.
3. Remove from heat and stir in remaining ingredients. Allow to cool slightly.
4. Spoon about 3 tablespoon of mixture at a time onto wax paper and press lightly to form a cookie shape. Chill until firm.

Per Cookie
Calories: 181 | Fat: 8g | Sodium: 55mg | Fiber: 2g | Protein: 4g

Cheater's Pumpkin Pie Cupcakes

Add a handful of raisins or chopped walnuts if you'd like a little texture, or frost and garnish with fall-colored vegan candies.

YIELDS 1 DOZEN CUPCAKES

1 box vegan spice cake or yellow cake mix

1 (16-ounce) can pumpkin purée

¼ cup soymilk

½ teaspoon pumpkin pie spice (if using yellow cake mix only)

Folic Acid: only present in very small amounts

Vitamin B$_{12}$: 🍎

Protein: 🍎

Iron: 🍎

Zinc: only present in very small amounts

Calcium: 🍎

Vitamin D: only present in very small amounts

1. Preheat oven according to instructions on cake mix package and lightly grease or line a muffin tin.
2. Combine all ingredients in a large bowl.
3. Fill cupcakes about two-thirds full and bake according to instructions on cake mix.

Per Cupcake
Calories: 195 | Fat: 3g | Sodium: 284mg | Fiber: 1g | Protein: 3g

Chocolate Cheater's Cupcakes

Use a vegan chocolate cake mix and add 1½ tablespoons of cocoa powder. Kick it up a notch with a handful of vegan chocolate chips.

"Secret Ingredient" Cake Mix Cake

This is another one of those unbelievable recipes that only vegans seem to know about. You just have to try it to believe it! Top off this cake mix cake with either the Basic Vegan Vanilla Icing or the Chocolate Mocha Frosting found later in this chapter.

SERVES 8

1 box vegan cake mix

1 (12-ounce) can full-sugar soda (not diet)

Folic Acid: NA

Vitamin B$_{12}$: NA

Protein: 🍎

Iron: 🍎

Zinc: NA

Calcium: 🍎🍎

Vitamin D: NA

1. Grease your cake pan well, as the reduced fat in this cake makes it a bit "stickier."
2. Preheat oven according to package instructions.
3. Mix together cake mix and soda, pour into a cake pan, and bake immediately according to package instructions.

Per Serving
Calories: 289 | Fat: 5g | Sodium: 425mg | Fiber: 0g | Protein: 3g

Flavor Combos

Experiment with different flavor combinations just for fun! Try a lemon-lime or orange soda with a yellow cake mix, a cherry soda with chocolate cake mix, and a grape or strawberry soda with a vanilla cake mix.

Basic Vegan Vanilla Icing

This is a simple and basic vegan frosting recipe. Add a few drops of a flavoring extract or food coloring, or just use it as is.

SERVES 8

¼ cup fortified soymilk

⅓ cup vegan margarine, softened

2 teaspoons vanilla

3–3½ cups powdered sugar

Folic Acid:

Vitamin B₁₂:

Protein: NA

Iron: NA

Zinc: NA

Calcium: only present in very small amounts

Vitamin D: only present in very small amounts

1. Mix together the soymilk, margarine, and vanilla until smooth.
2. Slowly incorporate powdered sugar until desired consistency is reached. You may need a bit more or less than 3 cups.

Per Serving
Calories: 248 | Fat: 7g | Sodium: 111mg | Fiber: 0g | Protein: 0g

Frosting Tips

Use an electric or hand mixer to get it super light and creamy. Frosting will firm as it cools, which means also only frost cakes and cupcakes that are cooled already, otherwise the heat will melt the icing.

Chocolate Mocha Frosting

The combination of chocolate and coffee in a frosting adds an exquisite touch to even a simple cake-mix cake.

SERVES 8

¼ cup strong coffee or espresso, cooled

⅓ cup vegan margarine, softened

2 teaspoons vanilla

⅓ cup cocoa powder

3 cups powdered sugar

Folic Acid: only present in very small amounts

Vitamin B$_{12}$: NA

Protein: 🌶

Iron: 🌶

Zinc: 🌶

Calcium: only present in very small amounts

Vitamin D: NA

1. Mix together the coffee, margarine, and vanilla until smooth, then add cocoa powder.
2. Slowly incorporate powdered sugar until desired consistency is reached. You may need a bit more or less than 3 cups.

Per Serving
Calories: 253 | Fat: 8g | Sodium: 109mg | Fiber: 1g | Protein: 1g

No Egg-Replacer Chocolate Cake

Applesauce helps keep this chocolate cake moist without eggs or egg replacer and cuts down on the fat, too, and the vinegar helps to lighten it up a bit.

SERVES 8

1½ cups flour

¾ cup sugar

⅓ cup cocoa powder

1 teaspoon baking soda

1 cup fortified soymilk

1 teaspoon vanilla

¼ cup applesauce

2 tablespoons oil

1 tablespoon vinegar

Folic Acid: 🍎

Vitamin B$_{12}$: 🍎

Protein: 🍎

Iron: 🍎

Zinc: 🍎

Calcium: 🍎

Vitamin D: 🍎

1. Preheat oven to 350°F and lightly grease and flour a large cake pan.
2. In a large bowl, combine the flour, sugar, cocoa, and baking soda. In a separate small bowl, mix together the soymilk, vanilla, applesauce, oil, and vinegar.
3. Quickly mix together the dry ingredients with the wet ingredients, combining just until smooth.
4. Pour into prepared cake pan and bake for 26–28 minutes, or until toothpick or fork inserted comes out clean.

Per Serving
Calories: 213 | Fat: 5g | Sodium: 170mg | Fiber: 2g | Protein: 4g

Vegan Peanut Butter Frosting

You'll love this creamy frosting, and it's a nice change from the usual flavors, especially when paired with the No Egg-Replacer Chocolate Cake found in this chapter.

SERVES 8

1 cup peanut butter, softened

⅓ cup vegan margarine, softened

2 tablespoons maple syrup

½ teaspoon vanilla

2 tablespoons fortified soymilk

2 cups powdered sugar

Folic Acid: 🍎

Vitamin B$_{12}$: NA

Protein: 🍎 🍎

Iron: 🍎

Zinc: 🍎 🍎

Calcium: 🍎

Vitamin D: only present in very small amounts

1. Whisk together the peanut butter, margarine, maple syrup, vanilla, and soymilk.
2. Slowly incorporate the powdered sugar, using a little bit more or less to get the desired consistency.

Per Serving
Calories: 388 | Fat: 24g | Sodium: 257mg | Fiber: 2g | Protein: 8g

Chocolate Peanut Butter Explosion Pie

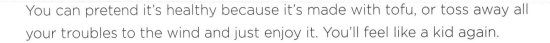

You can pretend it's healthy because it's made with tofu, or toss away all your troubles to the wind and just enjoy it. You'll feel like a kid again.

SERVES 8

¾ cup vegan chocolate chips

1 (12-ounce) block silken tofu

1¼ cups peanut butter

2 tablespoons soymilk plus ⅔ cup

1 prepared Vegan Cookie Pie Crust (see recipe in this chapter)

2–2½ cups powdered sugar

Folic Acid: 🍏
Vitamin B₁₂: 🍏 🍏
Protein: 🍏 🍏
Iron: 🍏
Zinc: 🍏 🍏
Calcium: 🍏
Vitamin D: 🍏

1. Over very low heat or in a double broiler, melt the chocolate chips.
2. In a blender, purée tofu, ½ cup peanut butter, and 2 tablespoons of soymilk until combined, then add melted chocolate chips and stir until smooth and creamy.
3. Pour into pie crust and chill for 1 hour, or until firm.
4. Over low heat, melt together remaining ¾ cup peanut butter, remaining ½ cup soymilk, and powdered sugar until smooth and creamy. You may need a little more or less than 2 cups of sugar.
5. Spread peanut butter mixture over cooled pie, and return to refrigerator. Chill until firm.

Per Serving
Calories: 561 | Fat: 32g | Sodium: 428mg | Fiber: 3g | Protein: 14g

Vegan Cookie Pie Crust

Use any kind of store-bought vegan cookie you like for this one: ginger-snaps for pumpkin pies, chocolate or peanut butter sandwich cookies for cheesecakes, or wafers for a neutral flavor.

SERVES 8

25 small vegan cookies
¼ cup vegan margarine, melted
½ teaspoon vanilla

Folic Acid: NA
Vitamin B$_{12}$: NA
Protein: 🍎
Iron: 🍎
Zinc: NA
Calcium: only present in very small amounts
Vitamin D: NA

1. Process cookies in a food processor until finely ground. Or, working in batches, seal cookies in a Ziploc bag and crumble using a rolling pin until fine.
2. Add margarine and vanilla a bit at a time until mixture is sticky.
3. Press evenly into pie tin, spreading about ¼" thick. No prebaking is needed.

Per Serving
Calories: 144 | Fat: 7g | Sodium: 228mg | Fiber: 0g | Protein: 1g

Pineapple Cherry "Dump" Cake

Just dump it all in! Who said vegan baking was hard?

SERVES 8

1 (20-ounce) can crushed pineapple, undrained

1 (20-ounce) can cherry pie filling

1 box vegan vanilla or yellow cake mix

½ cup vegan margarine, melted

Folic Acid: only present in very small amounts

Vitamin B$_{12}$: NA

Protein: 🍎

Iron: 🍎

Zinc: only present in very small amounts

Calcium: 🍎 🍎

Vitamin D: NA

1. Preheat oven according to directions on cake mix box and lightly grease and flour a large cake pan.
2. Dump the pineapple into the cake pan, then dump the pie filling, then the powdered cake mix on top.
3. Drizzle the cake mix with vegan margarine.
4. Bake according to instructions on cake mix package.

Per Serving
Calories: 498 | Fat: 16g | Sodium: 594mg | Fiber: 1g | Protein: 4g

Chocolate Graham Cracker Candy Bars

Matzo, saltines, or any cracker will work really well in this recipe, and because half of the candy bars will disappear before you're finished making them, you may want to make a double—or even triple—batch!

YIELDS 16 BARS

1 cup peanut butter or other nut butter

8 vegan graham crackers, quartered, or any vegan cracker

1 cup vegan chocolate chips

¼ cup vegan margarine

Optional toppings: vegan sprinkles, coconut flakes, chopped nuts

Folic Acid: 🍎

Vitamin B$_{12}$: NA

Protein: 🍎

Iron: 🍎

Zinc: 🍎

Calcium: only present in very small amounts

Vitamin D: NA

1. Line a baking pan with wax paper.
2. Spread about 1 tablespoon of peanut butter on a cracker, then top with another to make a "sandwich."
3. In a double boiler or over very low heat, melt together the chocolate chips and margarine until smooth and creamy.
4. Using tongs, dip each cracker sandwich into the chocolate and lightly coat. Pick up with the tongs and allow excess chocolate to drip off, then transfer to lined baking sheet.
5. Top with any additional toppings, and chill until firm.

Per Bar
Calories: 169 | Fat: 14g | Sodium: 156mg | Fiber: 1g | Protein: 5g

Ginger Spice Cookies

A delicious holiday cookie sweetened with maple syrup and molasses instead of refined sugar. Adjust the seasonings to your taste—add cloves if you like, or omit the allspice and add extra ginger.

YIELDS 1½ DOZEN COOKIES

⅓ cup vegan margarine, softened

½ cup maple syrup

⅓ cup molasses

¼ cup fortified soymilk

2¼ cups flour

1 teaspoon baking powder

½ teaspoon baking soda

½ teaspoon cinnamon

½ teaspoon ginger

¼ teaspoon allspice or nutmeg

½ teaspoon salt

Folic Acid: 🍎

Vitamin B₁₂: NA

Protein: 🍎

Iron: 🍎

Zinc: 🍎

Calcium: 🍎

Vitamin D: only present in very small amounts

1. In a large mixing bowl, cream together the vegan margarine, maple syrup, molasses, and soymilk. In a separate bowl, sift together the flour, baking powder, baking soda, cinnamon, ginger, allspice, and salt.
2. Mix the flour and spices in with the wet ingredients until combined. Chill for 30 minutes.
3. Preheat oven to 375°F.
4. Roll dough into 1½" balls and place on cookie sheet. Flatten slightly, then bake 10–12 minutes, or until done.

Per Cookie
Calories: 136 | Fat: 4g | Sodium: 178mg | Fiber: 1g | Protein: 2g

Cookies and Cream Cheesecake

Vegan cheesecake is a great way to dispel those stereotypes about granola-munching wheatgrass-sipping vegan hippies. Look for Trader Joe's brand chocolate sandwich cookies, Newman's Own Organics cookies, or use plain, mint, or chocolate Oreos, which may not be healthy, but are absolutely vegan!

SERVES 6

¼ cup soymilk

1 tablespoon cornstarch

1 (8-ounce) container vegan cream cheese

1 (12-ounce) block silken tofu

2 tablespoons lemon juice

2 teaspoons vanilla

¼ cup powdered sugar

¼ cup maple syrup

¼ cup oil

8–10 vegan chocolate sandwich cookies, crumbled

1 Vegan Cookie Pie Crust (see recipe in this chapter)

Folic Acid: only present in very small amounts

Vitamin B$_{12}$: 🍎

Protein: 🍎

Iron: 🍎

Zinc: 🍎

Calcium: 🍎

Vitamin D: only present in very small amounts

1. Preheat oven to 350°F.
2. Whisk together the soy milk and cornstarch in a small bowl. Using a handheld or stand mixer, combine the soymilk with the cream cheese, tofu, lemon juice, vanilla, powdered sugar, and maple syrup and blend until completely smooth. Slowly add oil on high speed until combined.
3. Stir in crumbled cookies by hand and pour into prepared crust.
4. Bake 40–45 minutes. Allow to cool slightly, then chill. Cheesecake will firm up more as it cools, so avoid the temptation to overbake.

Per Serving
Calories: 566 | Fat: 30g | Sodium: 597mg | Fiber: 1g | Protein: 6g

INDEX

About the Authors

Lorena Novak Bull, RD, has spent the last seventeen years working as a registered dietitian in public health and has more than twenty-five years of experience with vegetarian, vegan, and raw vegan lifestyles. She is the author of *The Everything® Vegan Baking Cookbook*. She is a member of the American Dietetic Association and a past president of the Inland District Dietetic Association. She lives in Riverside, CA.

Jolinda Hackett has been a vegetarian for nearly twenty years, and a plant-based vegan for nearly ten. She spent several years promoting the myriad benefits of a plant-based diet with vegan advocacy groups. Hackett has been interview by and appeared in *American Vegan* magazine, *Food and Home* magazine, the *Daily Nexus*, the *Santa Barbara News Press*, the *Jerusalem Post*, and on WZRD radio in Chicago. She lives in Santa Barbara, CA.